The Psychedelic Renaissance

Reassessing the Role of Psychedelic Drugs in 21st Century Psychiatry and Society

Dr. Ben Sessa MBBS BSc MRCPsych

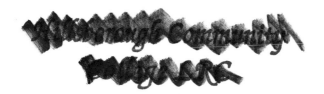

First published by Muswell Hill Press, London, 2012

www.muswellhillpress.co.uk

British Library Cataloguing in Publication Data

Sessa, Ben.

The psychedelic renaissance : reassessing the role of

psychedelic drugs in 21st century psychiatry and society.

1. Hallucinogenic drugs—Therapeutic use.

2. Hallucinogenic drugs—History.

I. Title

615.7'883-dc23

ISBN-13: 9781908995001

Printed in Great Britain

by Marston Book Services

*This book is dedicated to my children Huxley, Kitty and Jimi.
May your beloved pineal glands continue to secrete endogenous
mystical compounds forever more, giving rise to a lifetime
of spontaneous spiritual experiences.*

Contents

Forewords

Dr. Ben Sessa's insightful and comprehensive resource, *The Psychedelic Renaissance*, arrives at just the right time, when the general public is being increasingly informed by the media of the advances in psychedelic research taking place around the world. Dr. Sessa provides an in-depth, subtle, and reliable analysis of the state of the art of psychedelic research in the twenty-first century. With the wisdom of perspective, he also looks dispassionately at the excesses and mistakes of the 1960s psychedelic movement, and of the irrational and excessive backlash.

This is a book that deserves to be widely read. Dr. Sessa's *The Psychedelic Renaissance* prescribes a way forward for the mainstreaming of psychedelics and the many benefits they can offer when used carefully and cautiously, for a world in deep need of healing, spirituality and inspiration.

Rick Doblin
Founder and Executive Director of the Multidisciplinary
Association of Psychedelic Studies (MAPS)
May 2012

Psychedelic drugs are arguably the most important drugs for neuroscience. They produce profound alterations in many key elements of brain function such as perception, mood, insight and sense of self. For these reasons they have been used by different human societies for millennia. Currently, there is very limited use of them in science because of the intense regulations that control their production and use. These regulations are based on the false premise that psychedelics are extremely harmful drugs and are therefore designed to reduce their use. In practice, these regulations have virtually eliminated research in this field, which is particularly disappointing given that we have a great range of new techniques for exploring brain function such as fMRI ASL and PET neuroimaging scanning. Hopefully, this new book will encourage researchers to work in this field, to the benefit of our understanding of how the brain works and, in the longer term, to the development of new approaches to psychiatric disorders.

Professor David Nutt
Edmond J Safra chair of Neuropsychopharmacology at Imperial College, London and
former President of the European College of Neuropsychopharmacology and the
British Association of Psychopharmacology.
May 2012

Introduction

Apocalypse, Now and Then

These are interesting times. Some may say apocalyptical. While every generation flatters itself to imagine this is true, our own moment in history does indeed
feel special, for we are witnessing the unprecedented convergence of a number of
major crises and threats to our way of life and our planet: global warming, multi-
continental religious conflict with impending nuclear threat, wars for oil, wars for
water, riots in the streets and the supposed 'collapse of capitalism' in the wake
of the global financial crisis. Meanwhile, half the world is withering into starvation while the other half — just a click of a mouse away — die from obesity. You
couldn't make it up.

Profound alterations in consciousness are thrust upon us through the unavoidable bombardment of technologies, which shrink our world and expand our minds
simultaneously. Culture is homogenised into an unstoppable snowball of simili-
tude, and televised foreign campaigns push for obligatory global democracy. We
sit and watch as Sharia law dictatorships are pushed aside to make way for exported
TV talent shows and other symbols of progress.

Alongside our unremitting striving to survive, and in the centre of all this turbu-
lence and uncertainty, stands the contemporary Western individual — overweight,
spoilt, media obsessed and bored — yet searching as ever for the answers to the
perennial existential questions of human life. Of course, there is no single agent,
political solution or religious creed that will save the planet or us from this seemingly inevitable destructive march. Rather, a united multidisciplinary effort or
combination of efforts is required. But while we sit and wait for the more learned
political strategists in the hallowed corridors of power to come up with the answers,
what can we do as individuals?

Probably the only answer is to be ourselves. But this is easier said than done.
Who are we, after all, but complex bundles of multiple experiences, products of
our genes, our childhoods, our conditioning environments and our wishes for the
future? Amidst the cacophony of divergent influences pulling us this way and that,
it is easy to lose track of who we are and where we are going. If only there were a
simple key to unlock the door, a magical elixir to illuminate the way forward and
provide answers to the multitude of questions we ask, both profound and banal.
Alas, of course, there is not. And if there were such a thing it would certainly not

be a mere drug. It would therefore be erroneous to insert the three little letters 'LSD' here, as an author on this subject may have done if this book had been written 45 years ago in 1967. Psychedelics will not save the planet or us.

What *Can* the Psychedelics Offer Us?

But this fascinating group of psychoactive chemical compounds, the psychedelics, as they are commonly known, *does* possess something intriguing, some important qualities we may be foolish to ignore. Psychedelic drugs are the subject of this book, and although they will not teach us everything we need to know about ourselves, they may offer a new and innovative angle from which to help us approach the same age-old questions again.

—These drugs are uniquely placed to assist us with these queries, partly because of the fundamental qualities of the psychedelic experience itself and partly because of the place the drugs occupy in the development of our culture. There appears to be, at the very core of the psychedelic experience, a spontaneous stimulus to explore fundamental human questions. To quote a famous psychedelic folk band, 'What is it that we are part of? And what is it that we are?'[1] And perhaps even more peculiarly — for those of us with an interest in neuroscience at least, if not also religion — another feature that frequently appears spontaneously again and again at the heart of the psychedelic experience is, dare I say it, a *spiritual* element and an undeniable capacity for psycho-spiritual healing.

As a medical doctor in the UK, with a traditional medical education and methodical approach firmly rooted in supposedly objective, evidence-based scientific rigour, I have an immediate distaste for pseudoscience. The very word *healing* bothers me. Throughout the development of my medical career it has been a word I associate at best with homeopathy and at worst with the fringe elements of the New Age movement. Because, strange though it may seem as a modern doctor, I have not been taught to heal. Instead, my education has trained me to recognise, categorise, alter and adjust the pathology before me. I can shift things around, eradicate, overcome and obliterate — do all I can to mask the pathogens when they appear.

But then things changed for me when I began to learn about the existence and effects of the psychedelic drugs. And, for the record, I am not talking about a eureka moment of personal drug use in which I saw the light and decided thereafter to dedicate myself to propagating the wonders of this magical panacea to all and sundry. On the contrary, my epiphany came slowly and gradually — in line with my methodical scientific approach — but it may, I wonder sometimes, have taken me to the same place as the hippies.

My hope is that this book may have a similar effect: to gradually, slowly and with judicious 'scientific' rigour present the argument that medicine — and in particular psychiatry — needs psychedelics. And, moreover, as I have travelled this journey, I have learned to place that word *scientific* also in quotation marks for the same reason that I used to shrink from my nemesis, healing. Through learning about the potential role for psychedelics in medicine, I have inevitably examined the current role of science in my profession and the human condition at large. And I fear that I have, on occasion, found the word *scientific*, too, to be equally uncomfortable when applied to psychiatry.

Defining Psychedelic Drugs

What is it that fascinates people about the psychedelic drugs? And how can we best define them? A clue to the many ways to approach these questions comes from the various different words that have been given through the ages to this class of chemicals.

Brain Toxins

Mainstream psychiatrists might define psychedelics as those drugs that cause an 'acute confusional state'; they are seen as exogenous agents, coming in from outside the body, to produce profound alterations in consciousness, induce perceptual distortions in all the sensory modalities and generate the classical hallmarks of an organic psychosis. This definition is reflected in the medical term *hallucinogen*, a name often rejected by modern psychedelic researchers, not only because of the societal negative connotations it carries, but also because, in reality, the perceptual distortions induced by drugs such as LSD are rarely true hallucinations in the formal sense of the word ('a perception in the absence of an actual physical stimulus'), but, rather, more often illusions, that is, perceptual *distortions* of a genuinely present stimulus. Further descriptions of some of these medical terms will be given later in the book as we explore the individual effects of the major psychedelic drugs, as understood not only by the doctors who fear them, but also by the recreational users who revere them. One way or the other the doctors' definition of psychedelics is generally one of pathology: psychedelics are toxins mangling the brain that ought not be there.

Sacramental Gifts

Another definition of the psychedelic substances is afforded by a cross-cultural examination of their role in human experience. For many people, psychedelic drugs are considered spiritual tools or sacred medicine used by non-Western cultures as part of their religious or spiritual practice. In this context, some commentators choose the word *entheogen* (meaning the 'God creators') in preference to *psychedelic*. We know of, and have isolated, a vast range of naturally occurring psychoactive plants, fungi and animal products, such as ayahuasca, psilocybin, ibogaine, mescaline and bufotenin. And ancient humans most likely knew of many more than we do today. Some scholars have claimed that entire civilisations developed in symbiotic cohabitation with these naturally occurring compounds, incorporating them into their religions, using the psychedelic experience to validate their ordinary human experiences and inform their spiritual beliefs. That today there is an inevitable interest in such archaic times is of no surprise to many people of our generation who feel we are teetering on the edge of a cliff of biblical proportions. We shall explore later in the book the role these drugs have played in almost all societies of the planet. In archaic times and in development of our modern culture, psychedelics have had their place in creativity and the arts before and since the 'turn on, tune in and drop out' days of the 1960s.

Alien Visitors

The stalwart Western psychedelic converts — those starry-eyed hippies (about whom we will hear a lot as I betray my ambivalent conflict with their values) — typically neither question nor criticize the psychedelic drugs. But, rather, they tend to venerate them and define them as sacramental gifts from the gods. Leary called LSD, variously: the key, the philosopher's stone, the chalice and the Holy Grail.[2] Some, notably the brilliantly verbose psychedelic commentator Terence McKenna, have postulated that the psilocybin 'magic' mushroom was, *is*, an alien being whose spores have been scattered throughout the universe on meteorites in a deliberate act of propagation by a higher intelligence. Imbibing the mushroom provides a lens with which to communicate with wider extra-terrestrial culture. There are growing communities of followers of psychedelic folklore, to be found in online forums throughout the internet world, who hold their mushrooms aloft as the saviours of our race, the only possible hope we have to reconnect with our archaic pre-technological roots and save the planet from destruction. Many people align the magic mushroom experience with nature, a return to the earth, communion with the trees, the eschewing of modern living and the rejection of technology. Alongside them, however, many other followers of post-modern psychedelic culture paradoxically advocate an embrace of ultra-high technology, of computers, artificial intelligence and cyber culture, envisaging these chemicals to be the organic tools with which we can finally transcend our monkey bodies and emerge into the computer circuits of a neo-twenty-first-century internet-connected world set for interplanetary exploration.

Dangerous Drugs of Abuse

But there are still further ways to define and understand psychedelics. For many lay people, these substances are nothing more than illegal and dangerous drugs of abuse — addictive compounds, not to be distinguished from cocaine and heroin. Many people — from the police, to politicians and parents — will frame drugs such as cannabis, LSD and ecstasy as singularly destructive, the cause of an individual's, if not the whole of society's, ruin.

The current system of illegality, the infamous 'War on Drugs', as it has been dubbed, will be discussed in much greater detail in a later chapter. Not only is it a subject of great interest to people within many varied strands of society, but the current position of drug prohibition also carries important implications for the topic of medical research. In exploring the question of 'are drugs good or bad?'

(a transparently meaningless question — one may as well ask 'are knives good or bad?', and then try slicing a loaf of bread without one), we are forced to examine some fundamental questions about the structure of our society and laws. Issues of personal and religious freedom, the right to make one's own mistakes and the thorny subject of the 'Nanny State' come up, not to mention the arguments made in some quarters that we cannot possibly continue with an approach to the policing of drugs that favours the mafia, criminalises the majority of the world's population, and creates and maintains financially and morally unsustainable social systems. The drugs issue causes a tremendous rift in what the authorities are prepared to say in private and do in public. Few other subjects beside of the legalisation of drugs call into question more vividly the conflict between a technocratic approach to evidence-based politics and the emotional response of timid politicians, a conflict perhaps reflected best by a current popular anti-War-on-Drugs group called simply The Elephant.

Research and Clinical Tools

The final definition that I would most like to convey in the course of this book, which is perhaps unsurprising, given my profession, is that the class of drugs we call psychedelic may, with utmost importance, be considered as viable clinical tools to improve the plight of patients suffering with mental and physical disorders. Beyond this application, these drugs might even have an important role to play as agents to help us improve our knowledge of neuroscience and inform our understanding of human consciousness.

However, getting psychedelic drugs to market as viable mainstream treatments for mental disorders is difficult, to say the least. Personally, I consider the historical association of these drugs with recreational abuse a tiresome irritation. The truth is that LSD and MDMA began their lives in and, in my opinion, *belong* in, medicine. But trying to convince the general public and the authorities within politics and medical research of this is an uphill battle. Large numbers of people who would usually have no interest in the rather stolid process of medical drug development throw themselves into this debate with emotionally-laden arguments, which threaten to undermine the scientific process and hamper what would otherwise be the simple presentation of robust evidence-based data. My general medical colleagues, for example, wishing to develop new lines of drug treatments for liver, heart or endocrine disorders, rarely stimulate the kinds of hot-headed debate we see in psychedelic research. This may not seem unusual for those who cannot detach from what appears to them as the obvious fact that 'drugs like LSD are bad for you'. But from an objective scientific and, crucially, *clinical* point of view, it is most frustrating. So in this respect, the hippies, and their wanton advertisement of chemically-induced utopia through the use of psychedelics, have almost (albeit inadvertently) ruined the party for psychiatric research. For this reason, I feel continually inclined to distance myself from them in all aspects of my work with psychedelic drugs.

The Joy of Hippie Culture

On the other hand (and here is where my personal love-hate relationship with the hippies comes to the fore), as a cohort of recreational drug users, the psychedelic community is fascinating; they are completely unlike any other group of people who use drugs and about as far as it is possible to be from those who cite alcohol as their intoxicant of choice. Psychedelic conferences, those small niche psychedelic festivals, get-togethers and scientific meetings on the subject, are not hedonistic events. Rather, they are a colourful celebration of all the best aspects of reflective communalism, ecological thinking and harmony of shared differences. The majority of serious users of psychedelic drugs are uniquely respectful and understanding of their drugs' powers and dangers. They use the substances for healing (there's that word again), to search for a deeper personal understanding of their internal and external worlds, and to bring themselves and their families closer together. The psychedelic community is almost always closely linked with wider societal and global issues — especially those pertaining to the abuse of nature — and they often display an interesting mixture of extreme liberalism, a conservative appreciation of nature and a tangible humility regarding the human's place upon the planet. But, above all, a gathering of psychedelically inclined individuals is always a colourful celebration of the art, music and creative expression that flows from the psychedelic experience. It is hard to imagine a similarly enlightened or enlightening mind-set emerging from an annual conference of cocaine or heroin users — or even alcohol, for that matter, which, at best, would be a chaotic festival of self-serving egocentricity and, at worst, involve serious casualties and death. The reason for the difference between these groups of drug users is complex and encompasses many aspects of our cultural development over the last fifty years. But the chief explanation for the disparity lies in the fundamental nature of the drug experience itself. And it is this clinical effect, which, as a professional neuroscientist, interests me the most.

There are, then, many different ways to look at psychedelic drugs in these special and interesting times. When faced with so many conflicting environmental influences, it takes a novel approach and a willingness to go both outside and inside our heads, as it were, to help us to come up with some new answers to old questions. In these fascinating times we are now seeing many disparate elements of society glancing 'back to the future', looking again at psychedelics. Whether one aligns oneself with the doctors, the politicians, police, artists, the ravers, the hippies or the worried parents influenced by a dynamic but fragile popular media, we are in the midst of what I am calling a *Psychedelic Renaissance.*

CHAPTER 1

Personal Reflection

The literary world of psychedelic drugs is peppered with pseudo-scientific personal reflections. This is understandable: the experience itself is such a massive departure from everyday life — perhaps *the greatest* departure imaginable — that, once glimpsed, it is hard not to talk about it. In this respect, the experience has a lot in common with reports of born-again religious experiences, which can sometimes be painfully dull for the listener. But a new convert to religion cannot help telling all and sundry about it, even though their audience may not appreciate their words, such is the ineffability of their experience. For this reason, I wish to avoid any such verbiage. On the other hand, what I cannot say is 'I will stick entirely to the scientific point'. Because the truth is, from a scientific as much as from an epistemological point of view, that these substances are far from adequately understood by any discipline at this time. So, in order to justify why I am willing to base my judgment partly on subjective and unproved descriptions of these drugs, I would like to begin with a brief description of the journey that brought me to the study of psychedelics as a medical doctor.

Just Missed the Sixties

Apart from the occasional dose of cough medicine, no drugs of any kind featured in my childhood. Born just after the sixties, the youngest of six, I looked up to a family of older siblings who had lived through the height of the hippie counterculture. My parents were teachers and Quakers: my father a headmaster and English teacher who had emigrated from America, and my mother English. The household was libertarian, and I was brought up surrounded by the middle-class intellectual left-wing values of peace, pacifism and protest. From my older brothers and sisters I inherited an abundance of sixties records: Dylan, The Rolling Stones, The Beatles and Hendrix. Through my father I was exposed to Hardy, Lawrence, Kerouac, Huxley, Koestler and Kafka — and through them in turn to Ginsberg, Kesey, Laing and Leary. My mother gave me unconditional love, taught me to play music and inspired a passion for creativity, providing channels for personal transcendence and a boundless confidence to be myself. There was always a stimulating combination of live music, art and performance throughout my childhood. Little attention was paid to the television with far more interest in communal activities, such as making things and discussing ideas.

At 15 years old, I almost died in a climbing accident in Scotland, falling 60 feet off a cliff, breaking both my legs and lying on the rock face for three hours before being winched away by helicopter, then spending the next year in and out of hospitals and in a wheelchair. Thereafter, I developed a tremendous zeal for every breath of life, absorbing every precious moment of experience, fuelled with a sense of having been given a second chance that was not to be squandered. That experience also cemented my ambition to become a doctor, the first in my family amongst teachers, artists and musicians. In response to the pain I had suffered, I was determined, moreover, to be the first doctor who was nice to children.

From a Pair of Crutches to a Pair of Turntables

By the time I left school in 1990, 'rave' music had well and truly emerged into the forefront of contemporary culture, even in my rural Oxfordshire. Rave spawned the extraordinary summer-long scene of kids of my generation gathering in petrol stations that led to forbidden weekend-long parties in farmers' fields where they danced till dawn on a diet of cannabis, ecstasy and LSD. The summer of 1988 was dubbed the 'second summer of love'. Leaving this behind me, I took my guitar and set out on a six-month trip with two like-minded long-haired 18-year-olds to well-known hippie locations around the world: San Francisco, Hawaii, Australia, Bali, Thailand, Nepal. I read voraciously, and learned of the role psychedelics played not only in the formation of the drug culture of psychedelia, but in terms of the history before the sixties with the Beat poets and researchers like Kesey, Grof and Leary. I could see clearly that LSD and MDMA were much more than simply hedonistic playthings for ravers or hippies; rather, they were tools for psycho-spiritual development and, crucially, for medicine.

Studying to become a doctor was a dream come true. I dissected the human body and mind both literally and metaphorically through six years of medical training. This was coupled with the freedom of living in central London with other young people, DJ-ing and partying. I then took a year out and completed an additional psychology degree before finishing the medical course and eventually graduating to carry out clinical attachments in general medicine and surgery in Scotland. Once this was completed, I decided to specialise in psychiatry.

Mind Over Matter

For me, general medicine could not compete with the attraction of studying the brain, which is an infinitely more fascinating subject of study than any other (Woody Allen calls it his second favourite organ). At the time so much of the rest of medicine seemed, rather naively to me, like mere mechanics, whether it be blockages to tubes, breaks to bones or even chemical and metabolic imbalances in the heart or other tissues. But pure neurology was never much of a fascination either, as to be a neurologist felt like being a masterful piano tuner but never really listening to the music. No, the mental apparatus — and the human encounters its breakdown created — was the area that held the greatest appeal for me. Nothing else came close to the fascination of meeting people who had literally gone out of their minds.

Psychosis is always a big attraction for young psychiatrists, and initially I, like my trainee colleagues, thought this was the area in which I wanted to work. It is difficult not to be seduced by patients who believe their skin is blue, their brain waves are transmitted to Venus and the CIA are tracking their every move. But I soon found myself increasingly attracted to the plight of patients with anxiety and depression, and particularly those cases in which I saw people trapped in entrenched by earlier childhood experiences of trauma that had effectively stagnated their psychological development. Child abuse in all its forms cropped up again and again in almost every patient I met. During one of my attachments working with the elderly, I was amazed to hear 90-year-olds telling me about the pain of their relationships with their parents when they were just three years old, memories that never left them and have coloured every aspect of their life since. It is well known how those crucial early months and years of that bond between baby and caregiver set the scene for a future life of attachment with others.

I began to see little point in administering treatments to sick adults without first understanding for myself as much as possible about the beginnings of their pathologies, rooted in childhood, the place where the personality itself forms — and then often remains. Every book I read, from Freud to Laing, alluded to it. So, after twelve years of studying medicine and psychiatry in London, I made the decision to return to Oxford, this time to the university, to specialise in child and adolescent psychiatry.

Throughout my general training, I became increasingly involved in studying the history of psychedelics in medicine. I read everything I could find on the subject and pestered my tutors incessantly for the benefit of their experience and wisdom. Alas, no one could tell me anything about the potential for psychedelics as medical treatments. Some of the more wizened, bearded professors recalled a time when LSD gave a brief glow of light to clinical psychiatry in the 1950s and 1960s, but everything since then had been lost or forgotten. All my contemporary textbooks had to say on the subject was 'LSD: No medical uses' or they had extensive chapters on topics such as 'how to treat a medical emergency when someone has consumed a dangerous hallucinogen'.

Where Did All the Flowers Go?

But I knew from my private study that these drugs could be used safely and that there was a rich history of psychedelic research from forty years earlier. I devoured papers by the British psychiatrist Ronald Sandison and books by the Czechoslovakian researcher Stanislav Grof. But these names never appeared in any of my mainstream texts and, of course, even the well-known Timothy Leary, who I had always appreciated foremost as a clinician, was never to be found in the medical sections of the bookshops I frequented, though he could be unearthed — together with Grof and Laing — on the philosophy, popular psychology or even religion shelves. Frustrated at what looked like a deliberate whitewash, an attempt to eradicate this fascinating piece of medical history, I made it my intention to educate my contemporary psychiatric colleagues about the role LSD played, not just as a drug of abuse that influenced 'flower-power', but as a vital part of mainstream psychiatry in the not-so-distant past. I knew that for a brief time the medical profession truly believed psychedelics could be the next big thing to progress mental healthcare. I thought people needed to know about this part of our medical heritage.

Meanwhile, I was still learning the trade of clinical psychiatry and seeing frequently that the population of patients I was treating with traditional methods was often left wanting. I diligently followed the evidence-based algorithms specified by the textbooks and the National Institute for Clinical Excellence (NICE) that stipulated treatments with this drug and that — many of which worked for a large proportion of people. But I also frequently came across patients who, no matter what drugs or psychotherapy we recommended, were never able to connect with the cause of their problems, especially when it involved unresolved past trauma. Their ego and personality structures were too well defended, too strong for their own good, to allow themselves to break through and stare their childhood traumas in the face.

I looked at what Sandison, Grof and Leary were saying about this kind of resistance. They had talked extensively about the same population of patients I was meeting, comprised of people whose traumas were leaving them psychologically and existentially stuck. When LSD came along in the 1950s, these pioneering clinicians of their day had found, much to their surprise, that this peculiar new substance seemed to allow a special access to traumatic repressed memories. And, when combined with careful and diligent psychotherapy, the patient could be carried through the resistance to find some peace and resolution.

Ronald Sandison stumbled across LSD serendipitously while visiting the Sandoz laboratories in Basel in 1951. A year later he was giving his psychologically stuck patients the drug alongside their traditional psychotherapy, and finding the LSD increased their access to their repressed experiences. It brought into the open childhood memories, allowing the patients to concentrate on traumatic events of the past and providing associated emotional release. These people were desperate for this experimental new treatment. Many had been sidelined as hopeless cases, having had extensive electro-convulsive therapy (ECT), and were destined for psychosurgery if LSD didn't work. But despite their previous treatment-resistance, they were finding they now had a tool that enabled them to re-examine past relationships or behaviours. The drug appeared to provide access to a unique mental state, a *non-ordinary state of consciousness*, that under the supervision of their doctor allowed traumatic material to be worked through in clear, waking consciousness. Not only that, but LSD had some other unusual characteristics, producing in its users an intense flood of internal visual imagery, pictures in the mind's eye of both archetypal and highly personal recollections, a Technicolor route, as it were, to the unconscious. Furthermore, there was often a spontaneously felt sense of divine experience that allowed for spiritual growth and self-realisation.

Discovering the Lost History

Learning about the history of psychedelic therapy in the 1950s was an enlightening realisation of my own. Why, I wondered, had my profession turned its back on this apparently miraculous treatment? And why, forty years on, and with a dizzying pool of new medications available to the twenty-first-century psychiatrist, were so many patients from my own caseload not progressing? I knew Leary and colleagues were now seen as quacks by the orthodox psychiatric community, but there were elements of their approach that attracted me and I wanted to bring their methods back into the spotlight.

At the same time as I was learning from the past history of psychedelic medicine, I had also been following the beginnings of new research occurring in the U.S. In 1995 the Food and Drug Administration (an important American regulatory body that approves and monitors medical research) had granted permission for the first human study with a psychedelic drug, DMT, since the 1970s.[1] Increasing numbers of aging psychiatrists were emerging from the shadows to support revisiting research into the drugs psilocybin and LSD. And an American organisation, The Multidisciplinary Association for Psychedelic Studies (MAPS), which had been set up in 1987 in the wake of the emergency banning of MDMA, was now pushing vigorously for a new study to test MDMA's ability to assist trauma-focused psychotherapy.[2] All this looked like the verge of something new and vibrant in psychiatry, and a million miles away from the mainstream safety of medical practice in Oxford.

I looked up Ronald Sandison and went to meet him several times at his home. Then in his late eighties, Sandison was thrilled to learn a psychiatrist was taking up the mantle in the movement he started in the UK half a century earlier. He showed me old photograph albums of suited doctors and formal-looking nurses dispensing LSD to patients in the 1950s.[3] Although Sandison's work had attracted interest within the hippie community, until now no contemporary from his own profession had expressed an interest in rekindling his early research.

Turn On, Tune In and Disseminate

While learning from the past, I had also been following the beginnings of new research. Being in Oxford, it was only a matter of time before I came across the Beckley Foundation, Amanda Fielding's magical kingdom of consciousness research set in ancient rural settings.[4] Her lifelong dedication to altered states, propagating news of their existence to the masses and challenging the archaic laws that restrict these practices, inspired me to widen my net into the larger psychedelic community. In 2005, while I was still a trainee in child psychiatry, I wrote a brief report of what I had learned about this fascinating subject, which resulted in the first published paper about clinical psychedelic therapy in the British medical press since the 1960s.[5]

What happened next took me by complete surprise. Some of my colleagues warned me at the time against getting involved in this whacky fringe subject, calling it 'career suicide', urging me instead to choose a more mainstream topic for research, such as developments in antidepressant or antipsychotic therapy. In this context, I didn't expect much support for what I had written. To my surprise, however, I discovered a rich community of people interested in these substances, and I received invitations to talk at medical schools and academic gatherings of psychiatrists up and down the country. I sent my paper to Albert Hofmann, the discoverer of LSD, who replied with a positive letter of support and a photograph of him with his wife. I was discovering that there was a considerable network of psychedelic followers who, far from lying dormant, have been actively involved in propagating the message of these substances since the end of the sixties. But within British psychiatry I still felt like a lone voice — until, that is, I was contacted by two doctors from the Royal College of Psychiatrists Spirituality Special Interest Group, Nicky Crowley and Tim Read, both trainees of Stanislav Grof's transpersonal therapy. We put together a symposium for the college, entitled 'Psychosis, Psychedelics and the Transpersonal Journey', which was warmly received, swelled numbers further and put me in touch with an even wider network of like-minded people.[6]

Validation from Senior Figures

On finishing training in child psychiatry, I moved with my young family to rural Somerset to take up my first consultant post in which I saw a steady stream of adolescents with, among other diagnoses, treatment-resistant post-traumatic stress disorder. Meanwhile, I continued to gravitate towards academic psychiatry and published and peer reviewed more editorials on psychedelics. Professor David Nutt, the respected national lead for psychopharmacology in the UK, read my papers and invited me to talk to his department at Bristol University. Nutt was interested in encouraging the British government to review the erroneous and outdated classification scheme for illegal drugs that had been in place since 1971, and he had just published an influential paper on the subject, which, in particular, highlighted the relative safety of the psychedelic drugs.[7] I started attending his university department as a research associate. Around this time The Advisory Committee on the Misuse of Drugs (ACMD), which Professor Nutt chaired on behalf of the British government, was preparing a report about ecstasy, which was published in 2009. Nutt asked me to prepare a brief report about the therapeutic applications for MDMA. After consulting widely with experts in the field, the outcome of the ACMD review stated that MDMA was inappropriately placed in Class A of the Misuse of Drugs Act and ought to be moved to Class B, which better reflected its relative harm and safety profile.[8] An overwhelming wealth of evidence, including the plea that there may be a potential role for MDMA Therapy, supported this outcome.

Much to everybody's surprise and disappointment, however, the government disregarded the advice of its own committee and distanced itself from the outcome. Professor Nutt, the sort of doctor utterly committed to the scientific approach to the evaluation of drugs, objected to this blatant disregard of experts' unbiased opinions and published several protestations in the scientific and popular press. His efforts upset the British Home Secretary and eventually resulted in him being sacked from chairmanship of the ACMD. In an open published letter, the Home Secretary, Alan Johnson, stated that the then Labour government objected to Nutt, as an incumbent professional sitting on a government appointed board, 'lobbying for a change of government policy' and that 'it is important that the government's message on drugs is clear'.[9] How, protested Nutt, can the scientific, evidence-based truth be anything but the clearest message? His sacking cemented his position in the nation's consciousness as a crusader prepared to stand up to a government who disrespected their own appointed scientists just because they dared to clash with a pre-conceived, non-evidence-based political agenda.

All this was taking place while I was attached to Nutt's psychopharmacology unit in Bristol, and the camaraderie of his loyal department was tangible. I struck up a friendship with department Ph.D. student Robin Carhart-Harris, who I had first met a few years earlier at an LSD conference in Basel to celebrate the 100th birthday of LSD's discoverer, Albert Hofmann. Carhart-Harris was planning the UK's first human psychedelic drug trial since the sixties — and the first ever using the drug psilocybin, the active component in magic mushrooms. I got involved, helping out as the study doctor with some of the sessions and co-authoring the paper.[10] But more excitingly, I agreed to be the first subject in the study, which meant that when David Nutt injected me with intravenous psilocybin in the Bristol Royal Infirmary in 2009, I became the first person in the UK to be legally given a psychedelic drug for over thirty years.

Closure of the Past and Foundation for the Future

Since immersing myself in this vibrant community, the influence of figures such as Nutt, Carhart-Harris, Sandison, Rick Doblin of MAPS and the host of academic, literary and artistic folk I have met over the years has been immense. I feel a sense of closure in that these drugs connect so many aspects of my personal developmental history with my chosen profession. The experiences of many of my patients being psychologically stuck — just as Sandison had noted with his patients — and my glimpse of the clinical potential of psychedelic therapy are now too much for me to disregard. As we go into the twenty-first century, psychiatry is desperately in need of a renaissance. Too many of our treatments remain ineffective and psychiatric disorders remain unnecessarily treatment-resistant. In many ways the psychedelic drugs represent a real chance for a new way of looking at clinical treatments for patients trapped in intractable psychological conditions, especially if coupled with developments in the field of neuroscience, which is definitely the cutting edge of psychological research at the current time. Modern techniques for neuroimaging, which provide not only an anatomical picture of the brain, but also a real-time demonstration of its functional workings, are enviable tools of modern research that were not available in the 1960s when psychiatrists first discovered psychedelic drugs. Neuroimaging technology represents a massive potential for new research, revisiting those reams of studies of the 1950s and 1960s with new eyes.

My future plans include further work alongside Nutt and Carhart-Harris, as well as with colleagues from MAPS in America. I have a real determination to see the psychedelic drugs researched as potential developments for clinical practice. Despite my personal conviction about the potential value of psychedelic drugs, and although I know many of the public's beliefs about psychedelics are inaccurate, throughout my work I remain always cautious, aware of the controversial nature of the subject. My work in this field, I should point out is not driven merely by personal experience with psychedelic drugs, but, rather, by my experience with my patients. Post Traumatic Stress Disorder, which arises when a person has been exposed to a life-threatening experience that goes on to haunt them and cause serious dysfunction thereafter, is a devastating condition, now rising to epidemic proportions following the recent wars in Iraq and Afghanistan. I have watched helpless patients lose their battles with this condition and commit suicide, despite my profession's attempts to encourage them to access and work through their trauma. Psychedelic drugs are not a panacea, but I truly believe they could represent a potential extra level of treatment to help people who are unable to make progress with established forms of therapy, and that potential should not be ignored.

Undreamt of Possibilities for Therapy

In London in 1938, a year before his death and the same year Hofmann first synthesised LSD, Sigmund Freud wrote:

> The future may teach us how to exercise a direct influence, by means of particular chemical substances, upon . . . the neural apparatus. It may be that there are other still undreamt of possibilities of therapy.[11]

Freud was a neurologist prior to developing modern science's first systematic approach to the psychology of the unconscious, and I believe, had he known about psychedelics, he might have been a firm supporter of psychedelic therapy, recognising it as a vital marriage between psychotherapy and psychopharmacology, utilising a physical approach to directly improve his 'talking therapy'.

There remain many barriers to the acceptance of this concept. The idea that psychotherapy has to be hard work, and that drugs offering a quick fix or an easy pathway are inherently wrong, is endemic in psychotherapy. Carl Jung, Freud's contemporary (who, ironically, is embraced by the psychedelic community for his theory of the collective unconscious, which accords with many people's experience of psychedelic drugs) did not die until 1961, and he certainly knew about the psychedelic drugs. But he rejected them, saying the flood of repressed material in psychoanalysis was already sufficiently fast, and there was therefore no need to take a substance to increase it. This dogma — that the psychotherapy patient ought to be stone cold sober when he or she approaches their session — has persisted. But I wonder how many of these apparent cornerstones of traditional psychotherapy are also legacies of a Christian narrative that tells us there is something inherently wrong or immoral about the intoxicated state. As we shall see in later chapters, we in the West place a great deal of stress on the importance of being in control, and we assume access to the unconscious is best achieved with a sober brain. But this emphasis on conscious control is a very culturally bound phenomenon, specific to the modern West; it is a merely a matter of opinion, dependent on one's geography. And this belief is certainly one worth challenging if we are to explore all facets of possible treatments for psychiatry.

Indeed, there are many misconceptions to be challenged when one is involved in this work. I do not believe it is career suicide to do this work, but rather a ticket to an exciting future for clinical research. The field of psychedelic medicine may be considered an offbeat subject to those who find it difficult to unhinge themselves from those stereotypical images of stoned hippies dancing at Woodstock. But to those cutting edge neuroscientists at the world's leading research organisations, psychedelic drugs can no longer be ignored. They are becoming increasingly recognised as important tools to further our understanding of the brain. I would encourage any young and enthusiastic mental healthcare worker to familiarise themselves with research in this area. It could become an increasingly important part of the future of psychiatry.[12]

CHAPTER 2

The Experience and the Drugs

Why Do They Do It and What's It Like?

What is a psychedelic experience? What does it feel like? And why do people want to do it? These are very different questions to answer, and the second, for sure, is simply not answerable at all given that one of the defining features of the experience is its ineffability. The answer to the third question, why people do it, is considerably easier and is tied up in many reasons — some simple, some complex — to do with an individual's and society's needs. After all, one man's cognitive impairment is another man's party; there will always be plenty of good reasons for leaving all *this* behind and taking a sideways glimpse at life. Why limit oneself to just one normal waking state of consciousness? There were plenty of worthy commentators who consider it highly irresponsible for a person *not* to experience the psychedelic state — as grave a mistake as limiting oneself only to jazz or dub step and not even daring to try and listen to or rap or opera.

But what is the psychedelic experience like? Many artists, poets, musicians and literary folk, far more erudite than I, have attempted to answer this and failed, so I will not attempt an aesthetic appreciation of the psychedelic experience here. I could probably play what it feels like on the trumpet better than I could explain it in words.

Personally, I like Ford Prefect's description of another ineffable experience, hyperspace travel, to his friend Arthur Dent in *The Hitchhiker's Guide to the Galaxy*:[1]

Prefect: You should prepare yourself for the jump into hyperspace; it's unpleasantly like being drunk.

Arthur: What's so unpleasant about being drunk?

Ford: Just ask a glass of water.

Nothing can prepare one for what is by definition an experience that defies definition. One can read sentences like 'you become the essence of nature itself' or 'you become microscopically and macroscopically in touch with every living, breathing cell in the universe' or 'you experience all lives everywhere being lived simultaneously in the blink of an eye' — but what on earth (or elsewhere) does that mean?

Psychiatry — and, more specifically, psychiatric psychedelic research — has defined its own way of describing the state. There are a number of central features to the psychedelic experience, and many researchers and voyagers have tried to develop systematic schemes for describing it. Although no descriptions come close to knowing what it *feels* like, some of the psychiatric or medical 'mental changes' one can expect to occur after ingesting a 'classical' psychedelic drug are detailed below.

1. Physiological effects:

With LSD, from a physiological point of view, mild fluctuations in pulse, blood pressure and dilatation of the pupils are almost everything one can expect. If you want a drug with more powerful physical effects then consider alcohol. MDMA (ecstasy) or even cannabis may be a little different, with notable physical experiences of bodily relaxation. But, generally, the LSD experience is essentially a *mental* experience. Having said that, mental experiences can have *very* physical implications and associations. For example, after ingesting LSD you can imagine that your heart has stopped, your brain is leaking out of your eyes or that your kidneys now lie outside your body. These things don't happen, of course, but it may feel like they do. For an excellent description of this phenomena, as experienced vicariously through a dog, read Leary's account of a psilocybin trip he took with Richard Alpert in February 1961 in the book *High Priest*.[2]

2. Heightening or distortion of perceptions in all sensory modalities:

Under the influence of LSD, sounds may appear as more vivid, more 3-dimensional, as it were. The corners of the room no longer seem to meet at right angles; the walls seem to drip, breathe or flow with magnificent liquidity; colours appear brighter; objects may have an iridescent halo and everything pulsates as if alive. Tactile sensations become so intense that a massage on the skin's surface feels as if the bare bones themselves are being palpated.

And, of course, the sensory perceptions do not stay neatly in the modality that they ought to belong: sights can become sounds, for example, or a red flower can sound like a different tone of ringing bell than a blue flower. This phenomenon, synaesthesia, was employed by Owsley Stanley, The Grateful Dead's sound engineer and LSD chemist, who could see the waves of sound flowing across the stage so knew best where to position the band's speakers.[3]

3. Altered sense of space and time:

Time can move forwards, backwards or stay still. A lifetime can be lived watching the ignition of a match and then six hours pass with a turn of the head. Boundaries waver and then dissolve, eventually disappearing altogether. One's hand can appear to be ten thousand miles away from one's face and then all at once one is standing on the silvery surface of a grain of sand. Identity dissolves, one's sense of self dissolves. Clothes are seen as meaningless, amusing rags, as are the skin, the bones, organs or brain, and even ego and the self. One becomes simply a thought, a notion, an idea. And broader concepts such as society and social hierarchies are obliterated, prompting novel observations and new directions for thought.

4. 'Cinematographic' effects:

With one's eyes closed or if staring at a blank wall, one may be treated to a projected display of intense and vivid stories, an intensely personal or weirdly archetypal cinema spectacle of legends and flashbacks. Some have described this as a river containing all of one's experiences, as well as those of one's close family and distant relatives. One can reach out and manipulate the images, turn them around in space and explore their conceptual meanings.

5. Regressive behaviour and an increased recall of childhood memories:

In psychedelic self-exploration, every experience one has ever had is available to be looked at. The entirety of one's past is there, recorded, stored and waiting to get out. Under the influence of the psychedelic drug, as in dreams, its emergence may not be in its most realistic or obvious form, but rather as a display of latent and abstract images. Through careful attention, focus and practiced psychotherapy with a skilled facilitator this material may be interpreted and thus provide invaluable opportunities for self-discovery. There may be an accompanied rapid fluctuation of thoughts and emotions, which link the past experiences with the here and now. Like all features of the psychedelic experience, this increased capacity for recall can be frightening and overwhelming at times, which is why such care needs to be taken when using these drugs.

6. Increased sensitivity to the feelings of others:

Under certain circumstances and in some situations, such as with the high-dose LSD sessions described by Stanislav Grof or Christopher Bache, the psychedelic experience can certainly be harrowing, characterised by traumatic death-rebirth phenomena. But in less intense experiences there is usually an inherent peacefulness central to the psychedelic state. Many users find it difficult to experience aggression on MDMA, for instance. There is an integral sense of being with other people, feeling close to and understanding others' points of view. Empathy is a major therapeutic tool available through the use of MDMA, one that is well-recognised and an important part of it's therapeutic potential. So too, LSD was dubbed 'the love drug' in it's day, and for few years at least the hippie generation spread and advocated a culturally peaceful way of life. The fact that this was later poisoned in the context of twisted socio-political pressures was not a direct consequence of the LSD experience itself, but something altogether more complicated.

LSD is described by Grof as a 'non-specific amplifier', such that any emotion, good or bad, benign or destructive, can be magnified to dramatic proportions.

7. Religious or spiritual experience:

This aspect of the psychedelic experience has been studied extensively and passionately, and we will revisit it throughout this book. That psychedelic drugs induce feelings of spirituality, connectivity with God and an awe-inspiring sense of otherworldliness is undeniable; indeed, the associations of LSD with spirituality have been tested empirically on numerous occasions, from Walter Pahnke's famous Marsh Chapel Experiment in 1963 to Roland Griffiths' studies with psilocybin studies since 2006. And the role that psychedelics have played in the formation of many of the world's major religions is also well documented. Of course, the debate about whether the feelings of spirituality induced by psychedelics actually represent a true experience of God is sure to continue. Perhaps such questions can never be resolved, such is the nature of religious faith and spiritual experience.

8. Being at one with the universe:

Often called 'oceanic boundlessness', the psychedelic experience can trigger a sense of being part of a much wider entity than the traditional boundaries of personhood. One no longer defines oneself as simply a doctor, a father or mother, a husband or wife, a friend, neighbour or citizen; rather, one is a leaf on a tree, a drop of water in a lake, a breath on the wind. There is a plethora of vibrating energy moving like electricity through all things and one feels that one is part of it. One intuitively knows there is a cyclical balance to life that stretches back through time to the very origin of the universe and one is able to experience one's part in it. Paradoxically (to the rational mind), one may be as large as the universe and as small as the most elemental particle at the same time — everywhere and nowhere, inside and outside, alive and dead, timeless and historically rooted in time. Timothy Leary talked about the psychedelic trip as a cellular experience.[6] Using a rather beautiful language, he described how LSD connects us consciously with our DNA, allowing us to 'upload' information from our inherited genetic 'databank' and to relive memories of past lives, or to see and experience the lives of our ancestors. All this information, he believed, is encoded in DNA's double-helix structure that goes right back to the earliest amoebas swimming in a cosmic primordial soup, and that underlies the connectivity between everything. Scientifically, this reasoning is rather dubious (at least with our present knowledge about what is stored in DNA), but theoretically Leary's account is immensely attractive and Grof's research presents a similar view. Terence McKenna talked about a similar alternative universe, called 'the hyperspace', in which all space and time are stored, and which is accessible through the use of psychedelics.[7] Leary and McKenna suggest there is a kind of primitive primordial collective melting pot, which transcends the currently known laws of space of time but occasionally, under certain conditions, becomes accessible to us, illuminated by consciousness, and influences our lives.

9. Psychotic/delirious changes:

To many readers, much of the above may sound incomprehensible, like simple madness or confusion. Perhaps what I have described above is the result of pure suggestibility or even delusion, illusion and hallucination (symptoms often pertaining to psychosis), and therefore of no meaningful value and definitely not therapeutic — especially for someone with a pre-existing mental illness. I suppose it depends from which angle one is looking. Someone else may say the same about the rigid values and social structures we blindly follow, which to many people appear to be equally mindless and ill-thought-through.

There is no doubting — from whatever side of the debate on the usefulness of psychedelic drugs one is one — that the misuse of these drugs can cause harm. The depth and chronicity of the psychedelic experience can be frightening and disorientating for the user. For many ill-prepared users the experience is anxiety-provoking to the extreme. Feelings of panic and loss of control can overwhelm the user and in some cases lead to hospitalisation. And when these drugs are taken in non-clinical situations, without adequate support, by people with pre-existing mental illnesses these reactions can be exacerbated. This is especially true for people with a pre-existing diagnosis of psychosis. The concept of the 'bad trip' is well documented by both users and non-users of psychedelic drugs. The issues that increase or decrease the likelihood of having a good or a bad trip are discussed in greater detail in coming chapters. But what is for certain is that using psychedelic drugs can, for some people on some occasions, be a negative experience.

As a Neuroscientist, What Does All This Mean?

For all the diversity and range described above, one thing is for certain: the psychedelic experience gives one an entirely new way of looking at the day. From a neuroscientific point of view, what is interesting is that imbibing a drug like LSD makes one at least *think* these things are happening to one, which, for me, reveals something fascinating about the brain, especially if instead of simply dismissing these experiences as illusions, we take care to explore, map out and understand the neural and personal roots of such an experience. Then it really may have therapeutic value.

Another attempt at describing the qualities of the classical psychedelic experience comes from Bill Richards and Walter Pahnke in their 1966 paper 'Implications of LSD and Experimental Mysticism'.[8] I hope Professor Richards, who, from his position as senior psychologist at Johns Hopkins Bayview Medical Center, Baltimore, remains at the forefront of psychedelic research today, will support my paraphrasing of his words.

1. Unity

This aspect of psychedelic experiences refers to the sense of merger: Inside can merge with outside, self can merge with others, the Earth can merge with the universe, and so forth. Through these experiences of merger one can find an inner peace and unity.

2. Objectivity and reality

This involves the gaining of an understanding that one's existence during a psychedelic experience is real and that this feeling is itself genuine and valid. In the midst of psychedelic states, there is a sense that for the duration of the experience one can reliably answer that eternal question 'What am I?' with great lucidity.

3. Transcendence of space and time

This refers to the concept of losing one's sense of physical boundaries, one's ego and one's place in time. Those confining structures (time and space) become meaningless concepts as one merges with a wholeness greater than one's self. The everyday 'games' (as Leary called them) that constitute everyday experience become laughable distractions once the walls of space and time are stripped away.

4. Sense of sacredness

With obvious spiritual overtones this aspect of the experience refers to the sense of being 'overwhelmed by feelings of awe and reverence', or standing in 'the *white light* of absolute purity and cleanness'. Although such experiences may also occur without ingesting psychedelics, the fact that they occur so frequently when on these drugs sheds light on the close links between the psychedelic experience and the historical development of religious thinking.

5. Deeply felt positive mood

Simply put, this is the hoped for experience of euphoria, joy, pleasure, delight, rapture and sensual love. The psychedelic experience is, in Maslow's terms, a peak experience. It is a life-transforming ultimate experience in which the user soars with unbridled joy through pastures of ecstasy. While peak experiences can be both positive and negative, this aspect of the psychedelic state refers to the euphoric qualities of the drugs' effects.

6. Paradoxicality

This is my personal favourite element of Richards' list of attributes, for it describes the wonderful way in which the psychedelic experience can present one with such peculiar and illogical states of thinking even though they simultaneously contradict one another. For example: 'I am everywhere and I am nowhere!' or 'I am inside and I am outside!' or 'I am the size of an amoeba, I am as big as the universe!'. Such paradoxes appear strange and incomprehensible to the logical mind, but they make sense at the time, under the influence of a psychedelic drug. Ingesting the drug seems to bring to the foreground of consciousness a realization or insight that ordinarily remains hidden in the background of experience, unless one takes time to meditate deeply on the issue.

7. Alleged ineffability

As noted, it really is impossible to communicate the psychedelic experience to anyone who has not had an experience of their own. Unfortunately, this is one of those cruel twists of fate that polarises people into those who have and those who haven't. As Jimi Hendrix simply said in his inaugural album: 'Are You Experienced?'.[9] It also reminds me of the poor chap who, while high on acid, felt he had answered the fundamental question of the nature of life, the universe and everything, writing down his thoughts for many hours. The next day he searched for the scrawled papers and discovered all he had written was 'banana'.

8. Transiency

Needless to say, the psychedelic experience is not a forever experience — for if it were it would be incompatible with daily living. Rather, it is a special, sacred glimpse of the other-worldliness of the universe. A necessary part of the experience is that one must return back to normality, back to one's ordinary state of consciousness.

9. Positive changes in attitude and/or behaviour

This is a very important aspect of the experience, because although, as described above, it is ineffable, transient and somewhat illogical, nevertheless, once experienced that fleeting glimpse of he psychedelic state *can* result in important changes to one's self, one's relationships and one's entire outlook on life. Crucially, these changes can be real, lasting and positive.

The Importance of Set and Setting

A lesson learned very early on in the Western world's recent rediscovery of psychedelics in the 1950s and beyond is that the totality of the user's experience encompasses more factors than merely the choice of psychedelic drug used or the dosage taken. The concepts of 'set and setting' are essential, where set refers to the user's mindset, and setting refers to the environment in which the drug is taken.

Mindset includes a whole range of attitudes, beliefs and expectations: the users' expectations about what will happen, their experience of a particular drug, what they have heard from others, what the media tells them, what they know of the drug's physiological effects, what their fears and fantasies about what might happen are, what their religious orientation is, whether they wish to gain by taking the drug and what their past experience of mental states has been (both non-ordinary states of consciousness and issues surrounding their own mental health).

Setting includes the physical environment in which the drug is taken, who users are with at the time, what music is played (if any), whether they know the place, how hot or cold they are, how physically active or recumbent they are during the session, whether they have things to do the next day and even broader issues such as what is the social climate and attitude towards drugs in the environment in which they take them.

These factors, set and setting, have such a vast effect on the overall outcome of the psychedelic experience that they absolutely cannot be disregarded. When one hears horror stories of 'trips' that have gone wrong, it is invariably because of a lack of attention was paid to these factors.

Much has been written and spoken about what are the best conditions for a psychedelic experience. Leary's, Alpert's and Metzner's *The Psychedelic Experience* of 1964, which uses the framework of *The Tibetan Book of The Dead*, provides many useful tips on how to pay attention to both the right mind-set and the physical settings in order to achieve the best outcomes for a psychedelic trip.[10] Countless writers have since have expanded on how to get the conditions just right. Indeed, as a result market vendors over the years have sold many Indian print throws and incense sticks to countless students. The usual trappings of ethereal music and soft furnishing over which one can lounge are inevitable props. Many users will say these props are genuinely helpful, as they provide matching external stimuli for their internal mental state — indeed, they can encourage and foster a preferred internal state of relaxation. Similarly, many people choose to take psychedelic drugs outside in the countryside or in city parks, surrounded by nature in order to emphasise the often-felt connection with the earth.

Careful Planning, Due Care and Attention

The uniting feature of these settings is that the user must feel safe, free to express themselves and contained. Feeling unfettered by the annoying interruptions of everyday life is essential. Mobile phones or any other connections with the outside world are generally best avoided.

How to Take LSD Safely

It is important to engender a positive mindset before setting out on the trip. This is the case not just for the recreational use of these substances, but also when they are used medically. Indeed, it is something that all clinicians do with all their treatments. After all, when you go to your family doctor and she gives you a course of antibiotics obviously she doesn't do so in a malicious or hopeless manner. You would not leave her consulting room believing the drugs she gave you may cause you harm or even kill you.

Similarly, if you take a drug like LSD with the preconceived belief that it will make you go mad, cause you harm or ruin your life (which might filter through if you listen to certain aspects of the media) then the chance are you *will* have a miserable time. But if you have done your homework, prepared well and you take the drug in a relaxed and comfortable setting among people close to you, who you trust to look after you, then not only are you very unlikely to come to any harm (at least not as a direct result of taking the drug — of course, freak accidents or medical emergencies can happen any time), but you are also giving yourself the best opportunity to have a thoroughly magnificent and deeply profound experience. Indeed, when a drug such as LSD or psilocybin is taken under such carefully planned and judicious circumstances, there is every possibility that it will be one of the most important experiences of your life.[11]

In exploring psychedelics as clinical tools, the concepts of set and setting ought not to be seen as luxurious added extras or simple confounders. Rather, they are an active part of the experimental intention. The totality of the psychedelic experience is a combination of pharmacological and psychological factors interacting together in a synergistic fashion; set and setting are essential components of the psychedelic experience that *must* be attended to in order to achieve a maximum positive response.

Personal Opinion, Matter of Judgment and Disclaimer

Before I go any further, at this point in the book I want to be clear that I am not encouraging, supporting or condoning anyone reading this text who wishes to go out and take drugs, especially if that means breaking the law and especially if one suffers with any serious medical condition, including a personal or family history of severe mental illness. But what I am clear about is that if people are going to choose to use psychedelic drugs, then I urge them to do so with the utmost preparation. I am not a big fan of prohibition. Frankly, it is a waste of breath to tell someone 'don't take drugs'. The 'Just Say No' campaign simply does not work. After all, in the UK alone some 300,000 people take ecstasy every weekend and have been doing so for the last 25 years. Information is the essential feature people need to stay safe, and I will be pleased if this book can give people the necessary facts to minimize the potential harm of drug use. In later chapters, we will come back to the concept of harm minimisation versus total prohibition and discuss these in the context of the War On Drugs. But for the time being the most important message is Just Say *Know* To Drugs.

Personally, as both a brain scientist and someone with a personal interest in the expansive capabilities of my own mental apparatus, I would feel I had done my brain and my brief time on this earth a disservice if I had chosen to disregard non-ordinary states of consciousness. Psychedelic drugs certainly can be dangerous — Albert Hofmann, the discoverer of LSD and a fine proponent of its use throughout his very long life (he lived healthily to 102 years old) — was not shy of saying this.[12] These are immensely potent substances and they ought not be used lightly. With due care and attention, however, they *can* be used safely and they can very life-enhancing. But don't take my word for it, listen to the testimonies of the hundreds of millions of people who would tell you the same thing — if only they could put into words the ineffable nature of their experience.

Embracing the Challenge

The high-dose psychedelic experience is difficult, even painful and gut-wrenching at times (literally when one comes to ayahuasca). It is necessarily so. But what is so wrong with a little hardship and difficulty? Take the analogy of climbing a mountain or running a marathon. It would be foolhardy to attempt these pursuits without due preparation and care. Indeed, many hours of practicing, training and exercise are required to climb mountains properly. One must go into the activity with a positive mind-set, be surrounded by skilled guides, trusted friends and stable conditions. Even with adequate preparation, once the marathon or climb is underway it will be difficult. Sometimes it will be exhilarating and euphoric; at other times it will painful and challenging. But once one has reached the end of the race or climbed the mountain and come safely down the other side, one is often full of the joys of life, proud of one's momentous and perhaps life-changing accomplishment. Obviously, we don't advise people not to climb mountains because it is difficult or dangerous. We just caution them to do it with care.

Critics of this analogy might question how I can possibly compare the natural and skilled experience of rock climbing or long-distance running with the unnatural and indulgent drug-taking antics of a LSD taker. Well, firstly, who says psychedelic drugs are unnatural? And secondly, there is nothing *easy* about navigating an experience on 300 micrograms of LSD. Perhaps such critics are influenced by our Western world's ingrained narrative that there is something inherently wrong or immoral about non-ordinary states of consciousness. I believe this narrative must be challenged. Why is playing golf or watching opera any more natural than eating fresh mushrooms one has just picked off a rainy Welsh hillside?

As Donovan said in 1967: 'Don't do it if you don't want to, I wouldn't do a thing like that, oh no!'[13]

The Drugs Themselves

Classifying the Psychedelic Drugs

There are several ways of classifying and organising one's thoughts when it comes to the wide variety of substances available. The ranges of drugs I will cover in this section are not by any means exhaustive. Indeed, I will not be exploring in depth the ever-growing list of *Research Chemicals* (RCs) of which new ones appear for sale on the internet daily. These RCs can be bought — legally for the most part — with a mouse by any self-confessed drug geeks, who then swap the stories of their internal voyages on an exponentially expanding form of experiential drug blogs and tweets.[14] The RCs and all the political, psychopharmacological and legal wrangling that go with them deserve a volume of their own by someone with greater authority on the subject than me, so instead I will limit my lists to the more commonly known psychedelic drugs, mainly because the theme of this book is one of clinical medicine. Furthermore, the majority of those newly emerging RC drugs — some of which may certainly prove to be of clinical value in the future — are currently too recent to be considered for research studies. Most of the RCs, including the most well known in the UK, mephedrone ('plant food' or 'meow meow') have barely received even the most basic phase-one toxicology studies, and in that respect must be considered unsafe until more is known about their modes of action and effects on the human body. My advice is to steer clear of them. We have 60 years of reliable data on LSD — and yet still plenty to learn. One should obviously be wary of something cooked up last week in a test tube in a clandestine commercial laboratory in China.

On the other hand, skilled and diligent chemists can teach us a lot about the possibilities for continued psychoactive cookery. And for the world's most comprehensive guide to just about every psychedelic chemical conceivable, I direct readers to the chemist Dr Alexander 'Sasha' Shulgin's two books *Pihkal (Phenethylamines I Have Known and Loved)*15 and *Tihkal (Tryptamines I Have Known and Loved)*.[16] These incredible treasure-troves of psychedelic cuisine describe in great detail the psychoactive effects and the chemical construction of hundreds of substances from the very common to those so rare they are merely conceptual. In his books, alongside his recipes Sasha also describes some beautifully written stories about the last 50 years of psychedelic history. He has been dubbed 'the grandfather of MDMA' and remains a much-loved figure in the psychedelic world. I will return to him and his story later in this book.

Sticking, therefore, to the more common psychedelic substances, they can be organised according to their chemical structure or according to their effects. Looking first at their effects we may group psychedelic drugs into:

The 'Classical' Psychedelics

LSD
Psilocybin
Dimethlytryptamine (DMT)
Mescaline

The Entactogens or Empathogens

MDMA
MDA
2-CB
2C-I
2C-T-7

The NMDA-antagonist Dissociatives

Ketamine
PCP
DXM

The Kappa-Opioid Agonist Dissociatives

Ibogaine
Salvia Divinorum

We could also classify the same drugs into groups depending on their chemical structure. Most of the common psychedelics fall into one of two distinct groups. There are those whose chemical structure is based around the tryptamine molecule and those that are based around that of phenethylamine.

Tryptamines (or those psychedelic drugs closely related to it):

LSD
Psilocybin
DMT
Ibogaine
5-MEO-DMT
Bufotenin

Phenethylamines:

MDMA
Mescaline
MDA
Mephedrone
2C-B
2C-I
2C-T-4
2C-T-7

Close relatives of both tryptamine and phenethylamine are found in their natural states in high concentrations in our brains, which have lead some scholars to suggest the presence of endogenous psychedelic chemicals secreted by our brains under ordinary, apparently non-psychedelic, circumstances. For example, the common and immensely important neurotransmitter 5-hydroxytryptamine (also called serotonin or 5-HT) is the base molecule tryptamine plus an extra oxygen molecule in the fifth position of the benzene ring. The immensely potent psychedelic substance dimethlytryptamine (DMT) is simply the same tryptamine structure but with two extra carbons atoms instead of the oxygen. Both are extremely close to tryptamine structurally, but the effects on the brain between the two substances could not be more dramatic.

The theory is that these endogenous psychedelic drugs — particularly DMT — are released at times when we have naturally occurring intense, non-drug-induced experiences, such as religious, mystical or near death experiences. This is a fascinating possibility and intuitively it makes sense. Furthermore, the pineal gland is considered by many to be the site in the brain where the DMT is produced and released. Rick Strassman's work on DMT provides more detail about these ideas, which have not yet been established by rigorous scientific validation but are certainly worthy of further research.[17]

Some Common Psychedelic Substances in More Detail

1. LSD

Of the group we call the classical psychedelics, undoubtedly the daddy, or mother, perhaps, is lysergic acid diethylamide (LSD-25). Whether one is a fan of psychedelic drugs or not, one has to respect this substance for so many reasons: the manner in which is was discovered, the incredible effect it has had on the development of culture in the last 60 years, or simply it's pharmacology.

Pharmacokinetics of LSD

The compound has a plasma half life of around five hours and the experience lasts for between six and twelve hours, though some 'afterglow' effects can be felt for several days. The difference between the relatively short half-life and the lengthy intoxication itself suggests LSD may trigger a central psychological reaction that remains self-perpetuating long after the influence of the chemical itself has degraded. Users who are finding the going tough will be relieved to know that one way or another it will end eventually. As we have seen, the actual felt experience, described in detail earlier, is highly dependent on set and setting. A user may take a given dose in a given setting and feel virtually nothing or take the same dose under different conditions and have a very strong experience, which means there are many non-pharmacological decisive factors that contribute to the overall drug experience.

Pharmacodynamics of LSD

Although the classical psychedelic drugs influence many major neurotransmitters, the main psychedelic effects of LSD relate to its role as a potent agonist at 5-HT$_{2A}$ receptors in the layer IV pyramidal cells of the cerebral cortex.[18] The exact mode of action — how this effect causes the extraordinary mental experiences that occur — is poorly understood, though it is believed the effect is mediated through increasing glutamate release and associated excitation in that area.

Aldous Huxley, in his description of the effects of mescaline and LSD, talked of the so-called reducing valve hypothesis in which he proposed that psychedelics work by inhibiting the brain's natural tendency to block out a large proportion of the actual perceptual stimuli that that floods into it.[19] In other words, our brains act as valves and only present a small fraction of this material to our normal consciousness. As Huxley put it in *The Doors of Perception*:

> The function of the brain and nervous system is to protect us from being overwhelmed and confused by this mass of largely useless and irrelevant knowledge, by shutting out most of what we should otherwise perceive or remember at any moment, and leaving only that very small and special selection which is likely to be practically useful.

He said that under the influence of mescaline or LSD this mechanism is switched off and we are treated to an overwhelming cacophony of sights, sounds, colours and feelings — all of which are actually 'out there', but we normally do not get a chance to experience such delights.

Huxley was not a neuroscientist, but contemporary studies demonstrate that in some respects he was not far off the mark. However, breaking research on psilocybin by Robin Carhart-Harris at Bristol University and Imperial University has demonstrated that the classical psychedelics may actually have a markedly different effect on the brain, almost the opposite of Huxley's proposal.[20] That is, Carhart-Harris' functional MRI scans of healthy controls who have been injected with psilocybin demonstrate a *reduction* in cerebral blood flow, reduced glucose and oxygen consumption and an overall *decreased* functional brain activity. This would suggest that, rather than psychedelics 'expanding' our minds and opening up our conscious awareness to an increased, enlarged experience of external perceptions, the brain is put into a 'starved state', a 'default mode' state. Under this condition, one of two (or perhaps both) things may be happening: It may be that, without the internal reducing valve capacity, the external flood of perceptual information is allowed to come into our conscious awareness unchecked, thus presenting our consciousness with the kaleidoscopic display of 'what is really out there'. Or it may be that, when the brain is shut down in this way, we then *lack* sufficient external information coming in, so instead are treated to a kaleidoscopic display of *internal* imagery — all the top-down memories of the past are no longer held back and instead fill one's awareness. One way or the other, we certainly appear to experience life as 'if the doors of perception were cleansed'.

The latter suggestion — that psychedelics block out the external world and leave us at the mercy of our internal imaginary world — feels more intuitively correct to me, as one would assume the brain would require more, not less, energy to process (or even appreciate) external material. In other words, our brains use energy to keep the real world out. If so, psychedelics don't actually 'expand our minds', as we have always been lead to think. On the contrary, they may temporarily *shrink* our minds. This is an important distinction, and not one, I would imagine, that many psychedelic enthusiasts want to hear. As we have seen, trippers typically like to believe that the rocks and trees are alive, breathing with an intense inner beauty that the LSD allows them to perceive.

However this is not an issue that need reduce our appreciation of the psychedelic chemicals. On the contrary, as tools for psychotherapy the concept that these drugs can *force us* into our internal worlds is not bad at all. On the other hand, as I was one of the guinea pigs for Carhart-Harris' research, and some of the fMRI images that have been circulated with Robin's writings were of my brain, perhaps it is only me who has the shrunken mind.

The hope is that other studies of this type will continue to tell us about how psychedelics work, how the brain operates and, crucially, how we can develop medical treatments to help us use this information to improve the lives of patients whose struggle to manage their emotional memories is the cause of their suffering.

Dosage and Usage of LSD in Popular Culture

LSD is the most potent drug on the planet bar none. This colourless, odourless, tasteless substance has an effect on humans at a dose of just 20 micrograms, which is twenty millionths of a gram. An imperceptible grain of LSD on the head of a pin can alter the consciousness of a person for twelve hours and, as conspiracy theorists like to tell, a few well-placed kilograms in the water supply could incapacitate a whole city — although I'm not sure how well verified that urban myth is.

In the 1960s, the high doses were legendary. Initially, LSD was usually taken in a liquid form, dropped onto a sugar cube or some other delivery system. It was only available from the Swiss company Sandoz, where it had been discovered and manufactured for medicinal use. But by 1966, acid from Sandoz was increasingly difficult to obtain and underground chemists moved in to fill the gap in the market. Owsley Stanley III, the famous San Francisco chemist who produced millions of LSD pills for the burgeoning hippie culture, was proud to say he never dropped the bar below 200 micrograms. When Stanley was touring with The Grateful Dead in 1965, he met Tim Scully and the production got really serious. Between them Scully and Stanley put out one and a half million tablets of Purple Haze in 1966 and then White Lightening LSD tablets in 1967, which were carefully measured to be no less than 270 micrograms each.[21]

In 1969 Scully teamed up with Nick Sand, who was a member of the Brotherhood of Eternal Love, a global LSD manufacturing and distribution set-up, and this collaboration led to the famous production run of Orange Sunshine. In the UK, later in the 1970s, the alleged doses of the millions of LSD tabs made in London and in an isolated Welsh cottage, famously busted by Operation Julie, were at least 200 micrograms each.[22]

Most, if not all of the large LSD producers of the 1960s and 1970s were not in the business for the money. Rather, they rather saw their vocation as one of spreading the message around the world about this new substance, which they hoped would bring peace and harmony to millions of people. The doses were cheap (LSD in the UK was 50p a hit until Operation Julie put the price up). And LSD is not the sort of drug one throws one's money away on, repeating the experience again and again in an addictive fashion. Stanley, Scully, Sands, the Operation Julie mob, and many manufacturers and distributors since, have often given away at least a third to half of their LSD for free. This was not a business about making money — at least not for the chemists with their visions and values.

Today in the UK, the dose of a single hit of LSD (if one can find it, which is not easy) is usually between 50 and 100 micrograms. The most common form of the drug now is as a 'blotter', in which LSD has been absorbed onto a perforated sheet of blotter paper that is divided into hundreds of tiny single doses. The sheets are traditionally printed with colourful designs and (in their non-drug soaked form) often become extremely collectable, especially because they can be found signed by psychedelic luminaries of old and new.[23] Because of its very exclusive and infrequent pattern of use it does not carry much in the way of financial value for dealers to bother with. Indeed, for those who do distribute the drug it is often given away among a tight community of bespoke users.

Risks and Safety of LSD

LSD is a very powerful drug and can be psychologically harmful for people with pre-existing mental illness — especially people with a personal or family history of schizophrenia, for whom it could trigger a relapse or first episode of psychosis, which can be lengthy and lead to hospitalisation — although in reality such prolonged psychoses do not occur as commonly as they do when other drugs, such as the more potent dopamine agonists amphetamine, cocaine or even high-dose cannabis, are used by people with such a psychotic fragility. A more common adverse effect of LSD than a lasting psychosis is that the user may experience an acute unpleasant but short-lived event such as a seemingly unending experience of hellish visions and paranoid ideas, which they would wish to avoid in the future. But the risk of this happening can be minimised if the drug is taken with due care and attention and under the right circumstances.

From a physiological point of view, LSD is virtually inert. With hundreds of millions of people taking it worldwide consistently for the last 60 years, there have been no confirmed deaths from the physical effects of LSD. Herculean overdoses have been reported when people have accidentally taken hits in excess of 5000 times the normal dose, for example when mistakenly snorting a white powder assumed to be cocaine that turns out to be pure LSD crystals, but even under these circumstances physical reactions causing death have not been reported.

Of course, there are plenty of stories about accidents that can occur on LSD, which is why such care needs to be taken by the user. Yet these incidents do not come anywhere near the risk of accidents that result from the use of a drug such as alcohol. When they take LSD, the majority of people wander nonchalantly round fields or festivals or sit or lie very still as close to the ground as possible.

LSD is not addictive. Animal experiments confirm that it does not have anything like the abuse potential of drugs such as alcohol or cocaine. Rats in cages do not repeatedly self-administer themselves with LSD if given the opportunity to do so.[24] Humans reflect the low dependence potential for LSD in the observed epidemiological use too. Many people have experimented with LSD a few times, usually in their late teens or early twenties. The majority will say it was a positive experience but 'no thanks,' they 'don't want to do it again'. Some people will choose to be longer-term users and repeat the experience, but again the pattern of usage is usually very infrequent. Indeed, a 'regular user' may say they take LSD no more than once a twice a year or even less, but say they find it a fulfilling and positive experience, something to be shared with close friends and family on a social occasion. For the vast majority of users, the classical psychedelics like LSD and psilocybin are not the sort of drug one uses slavishly every Saturday night.

There are many misconceptions about the harms of LSD — as there are for all illegal drugs. In the late sixties, there was a rumour (based on a single uncorroborated poorly controlled and irrelevantly dosed scientific study) that LSD causes chromosomal damage.[25] It doesn't. Many scare stories at the time also circulated about certain acid causalities, such as the man who stared too long at the sun and went blind, or stories about people believing they can fly and jumping off buildings. It is difficult to confirm these stories, but what is clear is that when one looks at the relative risk profile against the massive pattern of usage LSD is a remarkably low risk drug. That conclusion may contradict media-driven preconceptions (or government policies), but it is the statistical fact.

Legal Status of LSD
LSD is illegal all over the world. It is a Schedule One drug in the USA and a Class A drug in the UK. Possession of any amount of LSD is a criminal offence and carries the risk of a lengthy prison sentence. Being caught and prosecuted for a drug offence is by far the most dangerous aspect of using LSD. It can completely ruin your life in a severity entirely out of proportion to the potential risks to your physical or mental health.

Potential Role in Medicine for LSD
LSD has a rich history of use as a substance to enhance psychotherapy for patients with a wide range of mental health problems including, in particular, anxiety-based disorders and addictions as well as possible applications for autism and neuro-psychological, social, or spiritual emergencies such as existential crises and end-of-life anxiety experiences.[26] The drug was studied extensively by the medical profession in the 1950s and 1960s before becoming popular as a recreational drug. It was subsequently banned worldwide in 1966, which halted medical research overnight but did very little to stop it's recreational use. All of these issues will be covered in more detail later on the book.

2. Psilocybin

Psilocybin is a naturally occurring classical psychedelic drug that can be found in many species of magic mushroom, particularly those of the psilocybe variety. In the UK the most popularly used magic mushroom is the *psilocybe semilanceata* — also called the liberty cap mushroom — whose distinctive pointy-headed appearance has become synonymous with psychedelic culture. There are hundreds of varieties of magic mushrooms, including the popular *psilocybe cyanescens, psilocybe mexicana* and *psilocybe azurescens.*

The magic mushroom has spawned generations of folklore tails, myths and legends — many of which are erroneous but have become ingrained into our social consciousness. It remains something of an enigma, with stalwart followers who often prefer its naturalness to the synthetic feel of LSD.

Pharmacokinetics of Psilocybin
The active component in the mushroom, psilocybin, is readily converted to the active component psilocin in the body, which has its effect on the brain in a similar manner to LSD, that is as an agonist at 5-HT_{2A} receptors.

Pharmacodynamics of Psilocybin
As with LSD, the effects of psilocybin are those of the typical classical hallucinogens. Some users will say they can easily recognise the difference between the LSD experience and that of psilocybin, whereas others, even experienced users,

cannot tell them apart at certain dosages. Interestingly, yawning — a serotonin mediated response — is a recognised common feature of the mushroom experience that one does not get so readily with LSD. As with all psychedelic drugs, the set and setting have such a significant effect on the overall experience of the drug's intoxication that it is almost impossible to create equivalent testing conditions.

In general, however, psilocybin is shorter acting that LSD; it's effects can be observed for a period of five to eight hours. Commonly, people describe the experience as 'slightly easier going', 'warmer' or 'more relaxed' than LSD. Again, however, there are many confounding factors as to why people may say this — perhaps, for example, it is a reflection of more commonly taking psilocybin mushrooms in a natural setting when they are freshly picked.

Dosage and Usage of Psilocybin
Magic mushrooms may be eaten raw and fresh, straight from the field, or they are often dried or brewed as a tea. The use of magic mushrooms is very widespread. For many people it is their first and only taste of a classical psychedelic drug.

As with LSD, psilocybin usage is generally not heavy or frequent for most users. Teenage experimentation is common, especially in rural areas in the UK, where for two months of the year it is almost impossible to walk over any patch of short lush grass without standing on liberty cap mushrooms

For liberty caps, which are tiny little things (the caps measuring just 10 to 15mm in diameter), a typical dose would be anywhere between 10 to 70 dried mushrooms — these figures representing a very low to a very high dose. Of course, many serious 'psychonauts' would call for higher doses. Notably, Terence McKenna talked about always consuming greater than 5 grams of dried mushroom as the gold standard for a psilocybin-induced mystical experience. This quantity is echoed by contemporary writer and mushroom connoisseur, Dr Kilindi Iyi, who can be found cropping up at modern day psychedelic conventions, such as the Breaking Convention, at which he described his high-dose psilocybin internal shamanic journeys ('alone in the darkness') accompanied by his plea that 'we need higher doses'.

Iyi is convinced that messing around in the foothills of altered states of consciousness is never going to offer one the degrees of insight that can be achieved by taking oneself into the stratosphere, so to speak. And the only way to attain this higher trajectory is to push and push with the mushroom dose until one can go no further . . . and then go further still. He is not shy of giving the following advice: 'If you feel worried and think "I may have taken too much" then that means you need to take more!'

This may sound like a rather reckless approach to some people, but I suppose when one is working with a drug with a virtually zero physical toxicity profile one can afford to push oneself with gigantic doses, assuming one feels psychologically robust enough to do so.

Risks and Safety of Psilocybin
Like LSD, psilocybin is virtually inert physiologically and recorded deaths from its toxicity are very rare indeed. Indeed, the lethal dose is over 1000 times the

usual dose taken for intoxication, which equates to having to consume approximately 17kg of fresh mushrooms in order to fatally overdose from psilocybin. This is unlikely to happen accidentally without the user having an enormous love of eating fungi.

However, unpleasant psychological reactions and accidents are far more common occurrences. As with LSD and all psychedelic drugs, paying careful attention to set and setting may reduce the frightening and disorientated effects of psilocybin. Like LSD, a psilocybin trip *will* by definition be a challenging experience at times. One should never consider entering into such an experience unless one is fully informed about the effects and has undergone thorough preparation.

One potential problem associated with psilocybin mushrooms is that of picking and consuming the wrong type of mushrooms. There are a number of causalities every autumn in the UK from young people who have accidentally eaten a poisonous mushroom that they wrongly identified as magic. Arming oneself with a colour photo guide to wild mushrooms and always having an experienced guide if deciding to go picking should protect against this. The wonderfully colourful book by Paul Stamets, *Psilocybin Mushrooms of the World,* is a good place to start.[27]

Legal Status of Psilocybin

Psilocybin, the drug, is illegal and is a Class A substance in the UK and a Schedule One substance in the USA. Possession of psilocybin can lead to imprisonment and a destruction of life opportunities in a manner that far outstrips any of the physical risks associated with using the drug.

However, the law becomes slightly ambiguous when one considers the fresh magic mushroom itself, which is effectively merely a vessel containing the drug. It has long been accepted that to prepare a magic mushroom in any way (which includes drying them or making tea) is illegal, but opinions differ as to whether it is illegal to eat them fresh from the ground. I hardly need to point out that if it is against the law to grow and possess fresh mushrooms on one's premises then the entire farming population of South West England and Wales would be liable for prosecution.

Until recently, for a few years in the UK there was a loophole in the law during which fresh magic mushrooms were sold in abundance on the internet and from many local markets using the legal defence described above. But this loophole was closed in 2005. As regards the current legal status, if in doubt, ask.

Potential Role in Medicine of Psilocybin

Psilocybin is a remarkably versatile and useful medicine for psychedelic psychotherapy. It has been used extensively in trials in the 1950s and 1960s, and is now being researched in many sites around the world for potential development as a licensed medical treatment. It has been chosen in preference to LSD for a number of the physiological, neuroimaging and clinical studies in recent years in the UK and USA, partly because it is slightly shorter acting than LSD and therefore easier to use with clinical subjects, but mainly because gaining ethical approval for use of psilocybin has been much easier than its more well-known cousin, whose very acronym tends to strike fear into the hearts of authorities, much more so than the humble mushroom.

Psilocybin has also been studied extensively for its use as an agent to induce a spiritual experience. This application is a reflection of its rich cultural heritage as a sacramental tool for many non-Western cultures throughout the world. We shall return to many of these uses for psilocybin throughout the book.

3. *N,N*-Dimethyltryptamine (DMT)[28]

Another classical psychedelic, DMT is an extraordinary substance in that, when taken by a human in its pure form, it is an extremely powerful psychotropic drug (one which has an effect on the mind). Yet, at the same time, it also occurs spontaneously throughout the animal and plant kingdom in a form that under normal circumstances has no mental effect on humans at all.

It rose to fame in the 1960s as 'the businessman's trip', capable of being enjoyed in one's lunch break, because when smoked it produces a very intense but relatively short-lived psychedelic experience, lasting just 15 to 25 minutes (though it may feel like several lifetimes). Today DMT is best known as being one of the active ingredients in the South American brew ayahuasca.

The intense otherworldliness of the drug's effects, and the very close resemblance between DMT and serotonin, has lead many researchers to wonder whether a great many of our everyday non-drug psychological experiences are actually mediated by a release of endogenous DMT.

Pharmacokinetics of DMT
Like LSD and psilocybin, DMT has its main psychedelic effects at the 5-HT$_{2A}$ receptor in the cerebral cortex, where it acts to restrict functional activity, thus switching off the reducing valve and providing to the user's consciousness a terrific flood of psychological activity.

Pharmacodynamics of DMT
The effects of DMT are similar to LSD and psilocybin in that the DMT intoxication may produce all the features of the classical psychedelic experience, including perceptual distortions, rapid fluctuations in thinking and, above all, an intense feeling of spirituality and connectivity with the universe. When the drug is injected or smoked, which delivers it very rapidly to the brain, users often report a powerful rush which comes on within 30 seconds. Not peculiar to DMT, but commonly recognised, is also the terrific sense of otherworldliness, including users seeing and interacting with 'entities', often reported as aliens. Terence McKenna described such interactions extensively with high-dose psilocybin (which structurally is closely related to DMT) and spoke about how his conversations with such entities support his ideas about the cosmic extraterrestrial origins of earth's psilocybin mushrooms.

It is always very difficult to ascertain the extent to which one person's trip report influences another. For example, there is now so much literature about the likelihood of meeting one of these DMT aliens that many users fully expect to — and then obviously *do* — meet one of the little green (or more commonly blue, interestingly) creatures when they take the drug.

Another area of science that has been historically connected with DMT is the phenomenon of the near-death experience (NDE). This is a massive topic, which we will not cover in detail in this book, other than to note that there are a lot of similarities between the psychedelic state and the NDE. Indeed, many scholars have proposed that it is during the throes of death, in particular, that the brain emits large quantities of endogenous DMT, to send us on our way as it were. Science has not come up with any substantial reproducible theories to explain what is happening with the NDE or how and why it occurs, but what is for certain is that it is a common psychological phenomenon. With over 15 million recorded occurrences, it is an area of science absolutely deserving of further research. Unquestionably, one's imagination is made of cosmic stuff; the human brain is amazing, and it can become tragically under-used and wasted if restricted only to the everyday waking state of consciousness. Much more research and field studies are required here.

Dosage and Usage of DMT
DMT has no effect if eaten as it is broken down in the gut by the enzyme monoamine oxidase. Therefore, it is not active orally unless also combined with a monoamine oxidase inhibitor (MAOI). For this reason, many users will either smoke DMT crystals in a glass pipe, or combine it with another smoking medium such as cannabis or tobacco, and smoke it in a traditional pipe. Either way, because of the route of administration the effects are always very intense and short-lived.

When DMT is taken orally, combined with a MAOI, as occurs when ayahuasca is consumed, the effects may be equally intense, though with a less sudden onset and, obviously, much longer lasting. We will come back to ayahuasca later in the book.

Pure DMT use is relatively rare. It is not the sort of substance your average drug dealer is likely to come across and certainly is not a big money-spinner for a dealer. But it can be found within established small communities of psychedelic connoisseurs.

Risks and Safety of DMT
As with other classical psychedelics, DMT causes a relatively minimal physiological reaction and therefore overdose is very unlikely, and no deaths have been recorded. However, as with the other drugs described the psychological reaction can be very intense and frightening without the proper due care and attention paid to set and setting. Another risk factor for DMT is that users without proper experience mess around with MAOI drugs, which, as all psychiatrists know, can be harmful substances if not prescribed and monitored with close attention.

Legal Status of DMT
As for the others, DMT is an illegal Class A and Schedule One drug. Possession risks imprisonment. The fact that it grows in abundance in every other blade of grass on the planet is another legal peculiarity.

Potential Role in Medicine for DMT

Our understanding of the role of endogenous DMT in mediating non-drug mystical experience definitely needs further investigation. DMT occurs in significant concentrations in many body tissues, but particularly in the pineal gland, which has lead some researchers to label this small gland deep within the brain as the 'spiritual centre' of our souls and DMT itself as 'the spirit molecule'.

In 1995, Dr. Rick Strassman led the first psychedelic drug human study in modern times when he investigated the subjective psychological effects of DMT injected at different doses into a small group of healthy volunteers. Results confirmed all the typical psychedelic effects, including the frequent reports of interactions with alien entities, who had something to say about the user and the state of the world. Rick Strassman went on to make some interesting postulations about the role of 'the sprit molecule' (the name of his intriguing book), which may or may not appeal to some readers, including speculations as to what role the DMT state can teach us about the presence of dark matter in the universe and whether there might be a cosmic connection between the recent observation that the foetal pineal gland begins emitting DMT on day 49 after conception and the ancient Buddhist belief that it is on day 49 that the soul enters the body.

This speculation aside, it is well worth a read and, above all, Strassman's study can be considered the first to pave the way for the modern renaissance of research interest. Strassman rightly concludes that it is difficult to see a role for DMT as a therapeutic agent, as the incredibly powerful short-lived experience under the drug does not leave a great deal of room for therapeutic engagement. But with a tool as commanding as DMT there may well be some other significant uses. The hugely positive influence of the ayahuasca experience as a therapeutic space is well documented.

4. Mescaline[29]

Mescaline is the last in the group we are calling the classical psychedelics. It is not a very widely used or well-known drug in the UK today, though it is used more widely elsewhere, especially in the States. At the end of the nineteenth century, it was the only widely known psychedelic drug in existence, and it has the claim-to-fame of being the first psychedelic to be recognised occurring in nature and then artificially synthesised. It is most widely known as the active component in the peyote (and a few other) cacti.

Mescaline is also well known as the drug that Aldous Huxley took when dosed by the British psychiatrist Humphrey Osmond in 1953 in the Hollywood hills.[30]

Pharmacokinetics of Mescaline

Like the other classical psychedelics mescaline exerts its main effects through its role as a potent 5-HT_{2A} agonist acting in the cerebral cortex.

Pharmacodynamics of Mescaline

The mescaline intoxication can include all the usual hallmarks of the classical psychedelic drug experience such as perceptual distortions, intense fluctuations in thinking and emotions, recall of past childhood events, regression, a strong sense of cosmic oneness, deep feelings of spirituality and a connectivity with every facet of life. Some users of mescaline will say there are less well-formed visual illusions or hallucinations compared to LSD, but more in the way of complex geometrical shapes and a greater sense of bodily or emotional changes, particularly those of a spiritual nature. But, as with all the classical psychedelics, the total experience is dependent on so many variable factors that it is often different to distinguish from the other drugs.

Dosage and Usage of Mescaline

While the commonest way of imbibing mescaline is through the ingestion of the cactus, it can also be synthesised and taken in an artificial form. In the UK, neither form is especially popular, and it can be hard to find outside of specialist circles of psychedelic geeks.

The peyote cactus itself grows extremely slowly. It has a green, circular, non-spiny appearance — the 'button' that sits on the surface of the desert with a pointed root below the sand. Traditionally, the buttons are cut off from the surface with the roots left in situ, then dried and eaten.[31]

The usual dose is between 100mg and 400mg (Huxley took 400mg), where one cactus button is equivalent to about 25mg. It is quite a feat, then, to eat enough buttons given their flavour. Many users say the experience is very long lasting and in particular takes a long time to come on. The main psychedelic effects are never-theless usually over after 12 hours, for the main part, although the afterglow effects, in which one can be left wallowing in a state of pleasurable inner warmth and existential well-being, can persist for over 24 hours.

Risks and Safety of Mescaline

Like the other classical drugs mescaline is fairly safe. It has only a very minimal physical effect on the body, even in very high doses. The risks are mainly psychological. As with other drugs, if it is taken without preparation the user may experience a state of panic or existential anxiety. The existentialist philosopher Jean-Paul Sartre is reported to have had an unresolved mescaline experience. Nausea is also a potential side effect of taking mescaline. But then these relatively mild side effects are unlikely to put off the serious psychonaut. As a famous psychedelic luminary once said, 'You have a tool to glimpse the secrets of the universe and you're worried you may throw up a little?'

But for those with a personal or family history of mental disorder (particularly psychosis), mescaline and all the other psychedelic drugs ought best to be avoided unless being used under strict medical supervision.

Legal Status of Mescaline

It is very dangerous indeed to have anything to do with mescaline or any other psychedelic drug because it is it is illegal. To be caught and imprisoned could cause serious and lifelong physical or psychological harm. However, there are some interesting loopholes regarding the legality of the peyote cactus, to which we will return later. In the North American Church, it is legal for registered Native Americans to use peyote cactus as part of their religious ceremonies, as they have been doing for thousands of years. The colonization of Native American territories by Europeans all but eradicated their ways of life and replaced peyote with the modern intoxicant of choice, alcohol, leading to hundreds of millions of alcohol-related deaths compared to the zero deaths recorded from mescaline use.

Potential Role of Mescaline in Medicine

Unlike the other classical psychedelic drugs, which have been studied extensively for their potential role in therapy, mescaline has received relatively scant attention by comparison. This may be because of its long duration of action that makes it difficult to use clinically. Or it may be because the drug is difficult to harvest and rarely synthesised, both naturally and artificially. Another possible explanation for why researchers have bypassed mescaline is that in the US, where the majority of psychedelic research has taken place, the drug is relatively well known and there is an established racially motivated socio-political opposition to the peyote cult. Or perhaps it is simply the case that no one has got round to it yet. One way or the other the field is wide open for clinical mescaline research.

There has been one notable study by John Halpern at Harvard Medical School in 2005 that looked more particularly at the epidemiological aspects of peyote use amongst the Native American population.[32] It is noteworthy that rates of alcoholism are considerably lower among those Native Americans who use peyote, which suggests there is further scope for researching the role mescaline can play as a tool to combat addictions. This is certainly an area worthy of closer inspection.

5. 3,4-Methylenedioxymethamphetamine (MDMA)

MDMA is not one of the classical psychedelics. Rather, it has been variously described as an *empathogen* or, by David Nichols of the Heffter Research Institute, an *entactogen*. There is an awful lot to say about MDMA. Not only is it a very widely used recreationally drug in the form of ecstasy, but it is also rising to the forefront as one of the psychedelic compounds proving to be the most useful as a tool to enhance psychotherapy.

For example, if one were to invent a hypothetical drug for enhancing psychotherapy what qualities would it have? It would:

1. Be short-acting enough for a single session of therapy.
2. Have no significant dependency issues.
3. Be non-toxic at therapeutic doses.
4. Reduce feelings of depression that accompany post-trauma (PTSD) presentations.
5. Increase feelings of closeness between the patient and therapist.
6. Raise arousal to enhance motivation for therapy.
7. Paradoxically, increase relaxation and reduce the hyper-vigilance that accompanies PTSD.
8. Stimulate new ways of thinking to explore entrenched problems.

These are all the qualities of MDMA when used carefully in a clinical setting.[33]

Pharmacokinetics of MDMA

MDMA works by stimulating a massive release of stored serotonin from vesicles in the pre-synaptic membrane, which floods the synaptic gap and transmits the nerve impulse to the post-synaptic neurotransmitter.

Pharmacodynamics of MDMA

As a psychotropic drug, MDMA has a remarkable and relatively rare characteristic, that of marked psychological consistency of effect. It is shorter acting than LSD (2–5 hours duration) and produces less in the way of perceptual alterations. When administered to healthy humans under medical supervision, MDMA is able to induce a mental state that is usually pleasurable to almost every user, almost every time. Apart from perhaps the opiates few other psychotropic drugs have this ability. While there is some anecdotal evidence that the intensity of the user's initial experiences with MDMA diminishes quantitatively with prolonged use, the qualitative experience remains reliably consistent. This consistency, together with our knowledge that MDMA acts as potent serotonin agonist, tells us a lot about the role of serotonin in mood states.

The remarkable subjective psychological effects of MDMA and how they relate so closely to the to 'the perfect psychotherapy session' are illustrated in the table below:[33]

Which Receptors or site in the brain?	What are the effects?	Why this helps with psychotherapy?
Increased 5-HT$_{1A}$ Serotonin 5-HT$_{1B}$	• ↓depression • ↓anxiety • ↓fear (at the amygdala) • ↓aggression and defensiveness • ↑self-confidence	• Less anxiety and aggression improves relationship with therapist • Allows patient to focus on trauma without being overwhelmed by negative affect
5-HT$_{2A}$	• Alterations in perception of meaning	• Facilitates new ways of thinking of old experiences
Increased Dopamine and Norepineprine	• ↑level of alertness • ↑arousal • ↑conscious registration of external stimuli (at LC)	• Improved behavioural readiness • Improved recall of state-dependent memories of stressful events • Provides 'Optimum Arousal Zone'
Increased alpha-2 activity	• ↑calmness and relaxation	• Provides improved mental state for exploring negative cognitions • Provides 'Optimum Arousal Zone'
All the hypothalamus	• Release of oxytocin	• Improved attachment with therapist • Improved empathy and closeness

Dosage and Usage of MDMA

MDMA is immensely popular (second only to cannabis) in the form of the illegal recreational drug ecstasy — or E, X, pills, gurners, disco biscuits, little fella's, smarties, beans, eckies, rollers, etc. I won't try to name them all; to do so will just show my age and not get anywhere near what the kids are calling them nowadays.

The drug is usually taken in the form of a white or brightly coloured tablet, often with a distinctive embossed design so users can compare batches. Pills are often called after popular brand names such as Mercedes, Mitsubishis, Ferraris, Volkswagens, Red Devils, Blue Nikes, 007s, Playboys, Batmans, Supermans, Rolexes, Pokemons, Red Stop Signs, Buddhas, Butterflies, X-Files, White Diamonds, Yin Yangs, Armanis, Doves, etc.

They are hugely popular, though their use is probably declining in line with a decreased purity of available tablets and a growth of internet-bought research chemicals. The average dose of MDMA in a street tablet bought as ecstasy is just 70mg, according to a recent study by Liverpool University's Dr. Jon Cole.[34] As well as, or instead of, MDMA, an ecstasy tablet can contain ketamine, caffeine, BZP, heroin, brick dust, dog de-worming tablets, methamphetamine, mephedrone, opiates, fish tank oxygenation powder or anything else that can be pressed into a tablet and stamped with a Mitsubishi logo.

As a result, many recreational users are nowadays turning to 'pure' MDMA bought by the gram, which they then swallow or snort. This practice, of course, does not guarantee purity, but rather puts the user at the mercy of whatever additional constituents their dealer has added to the powder. Ecstasy, which has been an integral part of the dance music scene for 30 years, is often taken together with other drugs — particularly cannabis and alcohol — but also frequently amphetamines and cocaine.

The sheer popularity of ecstasy makes clinical research on MDMA a terrific bind for those researchers who want to see the drug developed as a tool for clinical medicine. Of course, the doses, patterns of use and, subsequently, the risks associated with recreational ecstasy use do not equate at all well with the proposed clinical uses for MDMA. Unfortunately, the popular media and even some parts of the scientific community cannot separate clinical MDMA from its historical association with ecstasy. This obstacle needs to be tackled if we are to see the development of clinical MDMA in medicine.

Risks and Safety of MDMA

This is a necessarily long subsection as there are a lot of important misconceptions about the relative risks or safety of MDMA and it is vital these are accurately addressed with reference to contemporary research.

Using MDMA does carry a higher risk of physical harm than one sees with the classical psychedelics — no one will deny this. There have simply been no recorded deaths due to physical toxicity with the drugs LSD, psilocybin and DMT. But there are a notable small number of deaths each year attributed to MDMA. The numbers themselves remain extremely low given the massive uncontrolled use of the drug — some 100 million doses are estimated to be taken each year in the UK and the recorded annual death rate in the UK has been steady at around 20–40.[35] It may be that some users have a genetic predisposition to the potential harmful physical and psychological effects of MDMA, which then interact with certain environmental factors. More work is required to explore this phenomenon.

There are two major ways in which recreational ecstasy users can suffer acute (immediate) toxicity. The first is through hyperthermia.[36] This may occur through prolonged physical exertion in a hot environment, combined with dehydration due to not consuming enough water. The euphoric effects of the drug may lead to the user failing to notice the usual thermostatic cues and continuing to dance vigorously despite their rising temperature. The effects of hyperthermia include liver and kidney failure and cerebral oedema. Further serious complications include rhabdomyolysis and disseminated intravascular coagulation. High temperature has also been demonstrated to further exacerbate the risk of longer-term neurotoxicity.[37]

The second cause of acute toxicity is ecstasy-induced hyponatreamia.[38] In vulnerable individuals with a genetic predisposition for the condition, MDMA can cause an impairment of the kidney's normal water homeostasis mechanism via an increase in arginine vasopressin (ADH) that can lead to excess water retention. When this is combined with the potential for excessive water consumption (as has sometimes occurred because users have been over-vigilant about the risks associated with dehydration), there can be associated decreased serum sodium, which in turn leads to nausea, weakness, fatigue, confusion, seizures and coma.

In summary, then, when ecstasy is taken in uncontrolled circumstances, by naïve individuals, in extreme heat and with vigorous exercise, there may be problems associated with either drinking *too much* or *too little* water.

The other debate about the potential risks of MDMA refers to the chronic (protracted) risk of lasting neurotoxicity. Contemporary research on this issue has shifted the debate somewhat in the last ten to fifteen years away from concerns about lasting neurotoxicity. The vast majority of researchers today are accepting that at the typical doses used for low to moderate recreational use — and certainly at the very low and infrequent doses proposed for clinical use — MDMA need not be considered a dangerous drug.[39]

But there are some notable exceptions in the scientific community who buck the trend of the prevailing community. And their voice, which is often augmented by a vociferous media presence who have yet to get up to date on the contemporary data, add weight to the prohibitory stance against studying the drug on human subjects. This often restricts researchers to conducting their studies on either selectively biased populations of recreational ecstasy users (who frequently use other drugs or alcohol or have pre-existing mental health problems) or on animal models that translate poorly to humans and are irrelevant to those proposed for MDMA psychotherapy.[40]

The dose of MDMA given in the clinical context is usually a standardised 75–125mg, sometimes with a second booster dose of half that amount given several hours into the session. This is equivalent to around 1.0 to 1.8mg per kg.

In most of the current MDMA psychotherapy studies, the drug is only given once, twice, or a maximum of three times as part of a longer course of non-drug-assisted psychotherapy sessions, and there is always a gap of several weeks between the drug sessions.

When MDMA is given in these limited, infrequent and moderate doses the drug carries no risk of dependence, has no lasting neuropsychological or neurocognitive effects and no significant evidence of lasting neurotoxicity.

A study in 2003 by Schifano looked at UK coroners' reports of deaths attributed in part to MDMA between 1997 and 2000 and found 81 such deaths.[41] Of these 81 deaths, 59% of cases also included opiates and 60% included alcohol. Only 7% of those 81 deaths involved MDMA alone. That is six deaths in three years, after some 300 million ecstasy tablets were consumed by over a million people. And remember, these are *not* cases of clinical use of MDMA. These are cases of the recreational use of the street drug 'ecstasy' (whatever that is).

Given this data, it is clear that the media attention paid to the assumed dangerousness of MDMA is out of proportion. Even some of the scientific studies that have been historically cited a evidence for MDMA's neurotoxicity have either been methodologically flawed or bear no resemblance to the manner in which the drug is used by human populations.

For example, a study commissioned by the US government undertaken by George Ricaurte at Johns Hopkins University allegedly demonstrated severe neurotoxicity in primates given MDMA until it was discovered later that the bottles in the testing lab were incorrectly labelled and the animals were actually given the highly toxic drug methamphetamine instead of MDMA.[42] Ricaurte's paper in *Science* was subsequently retracted — though too late to have prevented the spread of an erroneous message about MDMA toxicity.

Other examples of when the results of MDMA studies had been erroneously used as justification for neurotoxicity in humans is when studies refer to massive doses bearing no relevance to human doses or patterns of use. For example, a 2006 study by O'Shea used MDMA doses on animals of 12.5 mg/kg — the equivalent of a human taking 12 and half tablets of street ecstasy.[43] And Hatzimitidou's 1999 study gave MDMA at a dose of 5 mg/kg twice daily for 4 consecutive days — equivalent to a human consuming a total of 40 tablets in four days.[44] And Sabol's study of 1996, which 'concluded neurotoxicity', was carried out giving animals 20mg/kg in repeated doses every 12 hours for four continuous days, which translates to a human being taking 20 tablets of ecstasy every 12 hours until they had consumed 160 tablets![45]

It is very bad science for people to make conclusions about the risks of neurotoxicity in humans based on this kind of irrelevant research. In contrast to these studies, a far more realistic study by Selvaraj that looked at brain serotonin transporter binding in former users of ecstasy as a measure of neurotoxicity found no such differences between ex-ecstasy users and non-users after 12 months of abstinence, suggesting any transient changes in serotonin neurons that may occur with MDMA use reverts back to normal after time, which contradicts the claims of lasting neurotoxicity.[46]

Legal Status of MDMA

When, in the 1980s, the rise of dance-music culture saw a shift of MDMA from the legitimate medical context to its use by a wider public, the drug took a path not dissimilar to that of LSD. MDMA leaked from the medical community and became the drug of choice for young people attending the rave scene. By the mid 1980s, there were increasing numbers of negative reports of its uncontrolled use outside of the clinical environment, and despite little evidence of harm the American Drug Enforcement Agency (DEA) called for the drug to be banned.

Those clinicians who had been using the drug safely and effectively for ten years requested that the case for medical applications for MDMA be heard, so at least the scheduling would reflect the calls for further clinical research to take place. This request was disregarded, and the DEA used emergency measures to bypass a hearing and make the drug a Schedule One controlled substance in the USA in 1985. This labelled MDMA as having a high risk of addictive abuse potential and no evidence of medical applications. Therapists were forced to give up using of MDMA, and the research collapsed overnight.

In the UK, the 1971 Misuse of Drugs Act (which had already been altered in 1977 to include all ring-substituted amphetamines such as MDMA, MDA, MDE, and the like) was further amended in 1985 to refer specifically to ecstasy, placing it in the Class A category.

Potential Role in Medicine of MDMA

The emergence of MDMA as an agent for psychotherapy can be significantly contributed to the pioneering work of the Californian psychotherapist Dr. Leo Zeff. During the 1960s, Zeff had been a psychedelic psychotherapist using LSD until it was later banned. By the early 1970s, he had ceased this work, but on discovering the psychoactive effects of MDMA came out of retirement and continued therapy with this new drug. It is estimated that by the time of his death in his seventies he had introduced (the then still legal) MDMA to over 4000 patients. Many of those who received psychedelic therapy under him went on to become therapists themselves.[47]

Largely based in and around California, from the mid 1970s to the mid 1980s there was a growth of clinicians using MDMA (then known as 'Adam'). Few published research trials exist of its use by therapists — and none that have the quality of double-blind placebo control — but there are many accounts of successful case reports and informal therapy outcome studies.

A paper by psychiatrist George Greer describes the therapeutic methods and the subjective reports of 29 patients who were administered MDMA as part of individual, group and couples therapy in the early 1980s.[48] There were no significant physical complications from taking the drug, and the overwhelming majority of subjects reported positive individual effects, improved wellbeing and the resolution of relationship problems after their therapy. In a later review of 80 patients who received MDMA therapy between 1980 and 1985, Greer outlined the careful methods and experimental techniques that facilitate a successful drug-assisted session. He also acknowledged the limitations of these studies, and suggested that further, controlled studies occur.[49] However the almost total prohibition of all MDMA clinical research that has occurred since 1985 has prevented such studies until very recently.

There are now a number of studies underway and (at the time of writing) one completed and published study.[50] Contemporary research centres around MDMA's use as a tool to enhance trauma-focused psychotherapy for the treatment of post-traumatic stress disorder (PTSD). This is an immensely important mental disorder to treat, especially as there are growing numbers of people suffering with PTSD. We will return to this in more detail in later chapters.

6. Ketamine

Ketamine is the last of the commonly used psychedelic drugs I will describe here. It comes under the class known as dissociative anaesthetics and it exerts its effects as a powerful NMDA-antagonist. Other NMDA-antagonist dissociative psychedelic drugs include dextromethorphan (DXM) and another odd substance, phencyclidine (PCP), which is also known as 'angel dust'. There is another group of dissociative psychedelics with a different mode of action, the kappa-opioid agonists. These include the active components from the plants ibogaine and salvia divinorum, which they will be considered in chapter seven when we look at some of the non-Western indigenous uses of such psychedelic plants.

A good word to describe the ketamine experience is *peculiar*. Its origins and place in medical history, public consciousness, and society is also weird; known to many as 'that horse tranquiliser' used by veterinary surgeons, it is also an incredibly useful anaesthetic agent for medicine, and indeed many paediatricians would feel unable to do their job if it wasn't for ketamine. Few other agents are as effective and safe as an anaesthetic than a brief shot of intramuscular ketamine when one is trying to relocate a dislocated shoulder of a howling child in the accident and emergency department. It is a lot easier to use and less risky that the equivalent high dose of benzodiazepines or opiates that one would need to get an equivalent analgesic effect.[51]

The reason ketamine works so well as a paediatric anaesthetic is the same reason recreational users enjoy its unusual effects. It doesn't work by simply blocking the pain receptors, as an opiate might (although it does do this to some extent), but it's main effect is psychological. It shifts the patient's attention away from the injury by presenting to them instead with such a peculiar mental state they forget their pain; it *distracts* the patient from their pain. Ketamine so effectively induces dissociation that pain gets pushed aside while the brain is side tracked by an extraordinary psychedelic world. In the context of paediatric anaesthesia, I have seen howling kids simply stop and stare in awe when that injection goes in. They look around the room with a puzzled look, fully conscious and awake but completely oblivious to the white-coated doctor grappling with their dislocated shoulder. Then, because of the short half-life, it quickly wears off and they can go home, without any of the hours of drowsy after-effects and risk of respiratory depression one would get with analgesic drugs such as opiates and benzodiazepines.

Ketamine is a synthetic drug, initially called CI-581, developed in 1962 by the pharmaceutical company Parke-Davis. It saw some medical use as an anaesthetic in the Vietnam War in the 1970s. There was some limited recreational use of the drug in the 1970s and some beautiful (and occasionally slightly chilling) accounts of it by the almost beyond belief psychonaut John Lilly. His story is well worth checking out: Be it his communications with dolphins, high altitude flight research, hours of high dose psychedelic sessions in floatation tanks with LSD, searching for extra-terrestrials with SETI or his methods for transcendence with ketamine, there is plenty in the writings of Lilly for any budding psychedelic enthusiast to get one's teeth into.[52]

Never gaining anything like the recreational popularity of LSD in the 1960s and 1970s, ketamine became popular as a mass intoxicant only when it was taken up by the later wave of the rave scene in the mid 1990s. It is that image of a wasted raver slumped in the corner in a 'K-hole', together with the horse tranquiliser adage that tarnishes ketamine and distracts people from what an important substance it is for clinical psychiatry and consciousness research. It seems that ketamine, like all the other substances discussed here, has its best days to come.

Mode of Action of Ketamine

Ketamine is a potent NMDA rector antagonist. (Note: we are talking here about NMDA, which stands for N-methyl-D-aspartate, *not* the drug MDMA!) The NMDA receptor is an important receptor in the brain that mediates its activity via the neurotransmitter glutamate. As an antagonist at the NMDA receptors ketamine inhibits calcium channel influx, which produces its analgesic effects. It is also this glutamate-mediated effect that makes it a very interesting candidate for furthering our understanding of psychosis.

Dosage and Usage of Ketamine

Ketamine is synthesised for the medical and vetinarial professions in massive quantities worldwide so there is no significant underground chemical synthesis of the drug. Most of what winds up being used recreationally is diverted from industrial production. In this respect, at least it is usually chemically pure. However, diverted supplies of the drug, when it has been produced in solution for injection, then get made into powder for insufflation (sniffing), at which point there are opportunities to mix the powder with other substances.

It may be injected intravenously, intramuscularly or subcutaneously. Recreationally, it is usually sniffed or eaten. Obviously, the former method of use produce a faster onset and shorter duration of action to when it is eaten, but in general it is not a long-lasting experience.[53]

When one takes a low, sub-anaesthetic, dose, one experiences the psychedelic effects. As well as distortions of perceptions and time, these take the form primarily of an extreme sense of disconnectedness with the outside world. People often describe an out-of-body experience, a sense of detachment and otherworldliness.[54] John Lilly and others have described very similar experiences to the classical psychedelics and spiritual experiences are common.

Risks and Safety of Ketamine

The truth is ketamine is not the safest of drugs. I know I contradict myself somewhat by saying that, as I have previously been at great pains to state that *any* drug can be dangerous and *any* drug can be used safely under different circumstances (and if this were not the case we certainly would not as doctors use so many highly toxic chemotherapeutic agents to treat cancer and as consumers drink coffee), but the problem with ketamine is that: a) it can be addictive; b) the acute intoxication itself can render a person vulnerable and, crucially; c) there are some worrying physical problems that can arise with heavy sustained use. Still, ketamine *can* also be an extremely useful and important drug when used in a cautious and careful manner in the correct setting.

The major physical problem associated with sustained ketamine use is the ability it has to inflame the bladder. A host of symptoms, sometimes collectively referred to as *ketamine-induced ulcerative cystitis,* include reduced bladder volume, pain on urination, abdominal and pelvic pain and incontinence. There have been many cases where such symptoms have remained permanently even after stopping the drug.

The risks associated with the acute intoxication are that the dose required for the pleasurable psychedelic effects is not too far from the dose required to cause total anaesthesia; thus ketamine can be referred to as having a narrow therapeutic window. Recreational users describe the wasted, zoned-out, semi-collapsed, speechless ketamine experience as a K-hole. This need not always cause serious casualties, because, as with cannabis, when it produces such intense soporific effects, at this point one tends to stop using it — being unable to actively dose oneself any further — and then the body gets a chance to recover. But there are serious risks of accidents when in such a state of high vulnerability, and especially so if one is injecting the drug.

A chilling account of such an accident involves the terribly sad case of the American Marcia Moore. She was an heiress to the Sheraton Hotel fortune and, like John Lilly, could appreciate the aesthetic, social and medicinal properties of such a unique and fascinating mental state. Moore wrote about her spiritual experiences with ketamine in a 1978 book *Journeys into the Bright World.*[55] But, unfortunately, the drug was also her undoing: she went missing one night in winter while partaking in a session of injecting herself with ketamine and was never seen again. Then, two years later, her skeleton was found crouched inside a hollowed-out tree in a forest near her house. It is thought she climbed into the tree and continued injecting ketamine, fell asleep and died of hypothermia. I have always found that image of a frozen skeleton sitting up a tree clutching a syringe to be very unnerving.

Another problem with ketamine is that it is also a relatively addictive drug. Chronic heavy users quickly find themselves stepping up the dosage to get the required effects.[56]

So, in summary, when one considers the risks of ketamine alongside the relatively safe drugs LSD, MDMA and psilocybin, with those images of addicted ravers lying in K-holes, incontinent with bladder problems — or, worse still, skeletons huddled in trees — ketamine has a rather scary edge. Certainly, it is a drug only to be considered with a great deal of care and attention.

Legal Status of Ketamine

Because of its wide and accepted medical uses, ketamine is a Class C drug (or Schedule 3 in the States), which is a very good illustration of the stupidly unfit-for-purpose classification schedule for controlled drugs. It has a much greater toxicity than the other safer psychedelic drugs described, all of which continue to languish in Class A and Schedule 1. But ours is not to wonder why nor question the wisdom of those in government who generously protect us with their drug laws.

Potential Role in Medicine of Ketamine

Apart from the well-established medical use in analgesia for minor surgery in emergency trauma, ketamine is also used an agent to induce anaesthesia for major surgery. Outside general medicine, however, there are also growing calls for its use in psychiatry. We will come back to this in more detail in later chapters, but, in brief, there have been some interesting studies recently looking at the role for ketamine as an antidepressant for both major depressive disorder and for treating depressive symptoms in people with bipolar disorder. Its role as an antipsychotic and, interestingly, its role as a psychotomimetic drug to help us understand better the process of schizophrenia, are also being extensively researched at present.

In summary, there is far more to ketamine than simply 'that horse tranquilizer'.[57]

7. Some Other Phenethylamines

It is worth briefly mentioning some of the 'newer' additions to the list of psychoactive phenethylamine compounds, which have emerged out of Alexander Shulgin's laboratory in the last forty years and were documented, together with the recipes to make them, in the book *PIHKAL*.[57] A number of them of have proved to be useful in (underground or unlicensed) psychotherapy, but there are no published studies of their use 'legitimately' in clinical studies to test them as adjuncts to psychotherapy. This does not men that they may not prove to be useful clinical tools in years to come.

Drugs in the '2-series' include 2C-B, 2C-T-7, 2C-T-2 and 2C-I. The one that has proved to be particularly useful for psychotherapy is 2C-B, often when combined with MDMA, because of it's relatively short half-life and ease of use clinically.

Mode of Action of 2C-B

2C-B does not have potent effects at the 5-HT_{2A} receptor like the classical hallucinogens and nor does it cause a massive release of serotonin like MDMA. Rather it may have it's principle effects at the 5-HT_{2C} receptor.[58]

Dosage and Usage of 2C-B

When 2C-B is used recreationally in the rave scene, it is often mistaken for MDMA. Many, but certainly not all clubbers nowadays, do not discern between one 'pill' and another, and may buy a batch of 2C-B and take them as if they were ecstasy tablets. The actual dose range is different from MDMA (usual recreational range for 2C-B being between 15 and 25mg, as opposed to five times that for MDMA).

Many recreational users describe the effects of 2C-B as broadly similar to MDMA, with more visual phenomena such as illusions, patterns and halos. Mentally, the user may feel an increased sense of awareness, energy and stimulation. Appreciation of music may be heightened. Many users say the 'come down' from 2C-B is easier going than MDMA.

Risks and Safety of 2C-B

As massive widespread use is not common, toxicity in the general population is rare. However 2C-B and the other 2C series of drugs have received relatively little in the way of toxicology studies and there have been some reports of death from it's use.[59]

Legal Status of 2C-B

Initially, 2C-B was not illegal. As with most newly synthesised compounds, they cannot be illegal until they have been picked up by law enforcement authorities and deemed as such. In the 1990s, the 2C-series drugs became increasingly used recreationally outside of the therapeutic context. 2C-B was produced for sale in head shops under the name 'nexus' and marketed as an aphrodisiac drug, especially in Amsterdam. It was not until 1994 that 2C-B was banned. It is now a schedule One (USA) or Class A (UK) drug. The other 2C-series drugs are also illegal in most countries now.

Potential Role in Medicine for the 2C-series Drugs

Myron Stolaroff, in his books *Thanatos to Eros*,[60] and *The Secret Chief* (the book he wrote about Leo Zeff)[61] describes the therapeutic use of several of the 2C-series drugs, particularly 2C-B. Taken as part of a long course of psychedelic treatments using many different drugs as adjuncts to psychotherapy, the 2C-series drugs can be beneficial tools for psycho-spiritual development, both individually and as part of a group.

The German psychedelic psychotherapist Friederike Fischer also describes her use of 2C-B alongside MDMA and LSD during her underground therapy practice in the 1990s. She considered it to be a helpful drug because of its 'unforgiving insistence'. She would only use it on those patients who were sufficiently orientated with the mental spaces created by MDMA and LSD. For such patients, it was a helpful substance to shift any remaining psychological resistance.[62]

There are, as yet, no planned clinical trials with these 2C-series drugs, though Stolaroff and others' experiences using these tools to assist stuck patients through multiple situations of personal and interpersonal crises provide powerful anecdotal evidence that they could play a role in the future of psychiatry.

A Brief Mention of 2C-T-7, 2C-I and 2C-T-2

TC-T-7 has a greater mode of action at the $5\text{-}HT_{2A}$ receptor[63] and is longer acting (8 to 10 hours, with a long, gradual descent) than 2C-B and according to Stolaroff has the capacity to reveal deep levels of personal awareness that may have use clinically. It is certainly not as popular recreationally, as it has a number of unwanted side effects, including sexual dysfunction, muscular tension and worrying cardiac symptoms in susceptible individuals. More study is required before its safety and efficacy as a clinical tool can be assured.

2C-I is known to have more psychedelic, as well as entactogenic qualities, at higher doses. *2C-T-2* has a similar mode of action and effects to 2C-T-7 and provides a powerful psychedelic experience.[64]

In summary, there are a host of established and new psychedelic compounds. As for all psychotropic drugs, they share similar core effects but also have marked differences. We have been so distracted by their recreational use that we have only begun to scratch the surface of the potential healing effects of these substances. In the next chapter we return to a time before such drugs were well-known and demonised by society.

CHAPTER 3

Early Pioneers of the First and Second Psychedelic Eras

In chapter four we will visit some mushroom chewing cave-dwellers and also a long-haired shaman from Galilee, but first we are going to jump to an important step on the timeline of psychedelia.

Historically, there have been three great eras of psychedelic culture. The first is centred on the dawn of the twentieth century; the second, and generally the most well known, incorporates the 'flower-power' era of the 1960s; and the third, well, that's the one we are rather excitingly in right now.

The First Psychedelic Era: 1880 to 1930

There was a stirring of interest in psychedelic drugs between 1880 and the 1920s, mostly centred on the drug mescaline. Hashish was also popular at the time, as was opium, which is not a psychedelic drug but its dream-like qualities were certainly responsible for many writers' creative meanderings.

People have known about mescaline, the active component in the peyote cactus, for a long time. But the credit for the first Western medical report on the psychological effects of mescaline on humans goes to the American neurologist and novelist S. Weir Mitchell, who, in 1896, turned his hand to describing the cactus in a paper for the British Medical Journal called 'The Effects of Anhelonium Lewinii (the Mescal Button)'.[1] Like so many others in psychedelic history, Mitchell was a colourful character. Prior to his interest in psychoactive cacti he had published works on subjects as esoteric as 'Gunshot Wounds and Other Injuries of Nerves' and 'Researches Upon the Venom of the Rattlesnake'.

His paper was followed a year later by two more from the British physician and psychologist Henry Havelock Ellis: 'The Phenomena of Mescal Intoxication', in 1897, and 'Mescal: A New Artificial Paradise'.[2] Havelock Ellis was another scientist with a broad knowledge base and an attraction towards atypical subjects. He also published what is arguably the first medical textbook on homosexuality and chose to lead a most unconventional life, writing extensively on the science of sex in spite of — or perhaps because of — his own unusual personal issues. He was a chronic sufferer of impotence and reportedly a virgin at the time of starting an open marriage in his 1930s with his lesbian wife. He was also reportedly aroused by urolagnia, which I will leave the reader to investigate.

Havelock Ellis and Weir Mitchell were keen proponents of the mescaline experience and their works inspired many others to explore the sensory and spiritual delights of the plant. A more scientific analysis of the peyote cactus had occurred ten years earlier by the German pharmacologist Louis Lewin, after whom the cactus was named.[3] Lewin was one of the first scientists to recognise the links between the pharmacology of different plants and their mental effects, and he attempted a classification of various different psychoactive drugs based on their psychoactive effects, bringing new words into popular usage. His categories included the 'euphoriants', such as heroin; the 'inebriants,' such as alcohol; and the class of drugs he named 'phantastica', which later became the psychedelics. Indeed, such was his influence that the words *euphoriant* and *inebriant* remain in popular usage today. In 1947, when Werner Stoll, Albert Hofmann's contemporary, published the world's first report of the effects of LSD he referred to Hofmann's new discovery at that time as a phantastica.[4] It was not until later in the late 1950s that the word *psychedelic* appears.

In 1897 another major breakthrough happened when German pharmacologist Arthur Carl Wilhelm Heffter succeeded in isolating mescaline from the peyote-cactus, which was the first time a naturally occurring psychedelic had been identified and extracted in this way.[5] Heffter's legacy is assured to this day by it being the chosen name of a contemporary scientific group at the forefront of modern research into psychedelic drugs.

The Second Psychedelic Era: 1938 to 1976

The discovery of LSD in the 1940s, and the days of early psychedelic research in the 1950s and 1960s, are well documented, with numerous psychedelic folklore stories of Hofmann's magical bicycle rides through the countryside around Basel. But some of the UK-based contributions to psychedelic history are less well known, although they have been described wonderfully by my friend Andy Roberts in his recent book *Albion Dreaming*, which is highly recommended as a description of Britain's part in psychedelic history.[6] And for those readers who have not already devoured every text available on the subject of the second psychedelic era, here is brief potted review of their recent origins.

Magnificent Realisations from Mouldy Rye

Albert Hofmann was a chemist working at Sandoz Laboratories in Switzerland. In the late 1930s, he was investigating a series of preparations based on the chemical lysergic acid, which is produced by the fungus ergot that grows on many different grasses and crops, but particularly on rye. Ergot (*claviceps purpurea*) was known to have psychotropic properties and was recognised as having been responsible for outbreaks of St. Anthony's Fire in the Middle Ages — peculiar epidemics of mass psychosis, hysteria and death when whole communities became poisoned by bread made from mouldy flour. But Hofmann was interested in another known property of lysergic acid: its capacity as a vasoconstrictor. He was part of a team of pre-war chemists and psychopharmacologists developing possible drugs to effect blood vessel constriction.

He diligently synthesised different combinations of chemicals based around the structure of lysergic acid and in 1938 produced the 25th in his series, lysergic acid diethylamide, which he called LSD-25 (the 'S' abbreviation standing for 'saure', the German word for acid — had the compound been discovered in an English-speaking country we may now be talking about LAD not LSD). It is widely believed that this moment in 1938 was the first time LSD had been brought into existence.

In 1938, before discovering its psychoactive properties, Hofmann then shelved his LSD-25. He did not return to it again until 1943, when, fuelled by a strange presentiment that it may have further use, he synthesised a fresh batch. It was dur-ing this process that Hofmann inadvertently imbibed a small quantity of the drug (probably by absorption of the crystals through his fingertips) and experienced a peculiar psychological episode characterized by dizziness and hallucinations:

> I became affected by a remarkable restlessness, combined with a slight dizzi-ness. At home I lay down and sank into a not unpleasant intoxicated-like condition, characterized by an extremely stimulated imagination. In a dream-like state, with eyes closed (I found the daylight to be unpleasantly glaring), I perceived an uninterrupted stream of fantastic pictures, extraordinary shapes with intense, kaleidoscopic play of colors. After some two hours this condi-tion faded away.[7]

What happened next sealed the fate of the psychedelic culture and spawned a massive body of new research. It is a direct result of Hofmann's inquisitive person-ality that history turned out the way it did.

Hofmann the Creative Explorer

Many other scientists, having experienced what Albert Hofmann did that day with his accidental absorption, might have either ignored it, brushed it off or per-haps labelled the tube 'toxic' and never returned. But for Hofmann, this was not enough. Always the exploratory scientist, with a creative imagination to boot, and a fascination for curious mental states, he decided to conduct a personal experiment.

A few days later, monitored by his colleagues he measured out what he thought was the tiniest possible amount of his LSD-25 — he chose 250 micrograms (a quarter of a tenth of a gram). The plan was to intentionally swallow this amount, which he did not expect to have any effect at such a small dose, and then slowly increase the dose by fractions of 25 micrograms until he felt something happening. For the record, 250 micrograms is a *whopping* dose of LSD — the average street dose today being between 75 and 100 micrograms.

What followed was another, even more intense experience and that infamous bicycle ride back from his laboratory to his house, where he lay on his bed. At first, he had a frightening experience and thought he was dying. His neighbour brought him a glass of milk and he thought her distorted image was that of a 'malevolent witch'. A doctor was asked to attend and was able to reassure him that all his vital physical signs were normal and he was not in any apparent physical danger. Then, as the hours passed and the intensity reduced a little, he was gradually able to enjoy the experience and drift languidly into hitherto unknown mental spaces of immense fascination and delight:

> Little by little I could begin to enjoy the unprecedented colours and plays of shapes that persisted behind my closed eyes. Kaleidoscopic, fantastic images surged in on me, alternating, variegated, opening and then closing themselves in circles and spirals, exploding in coloured fountains, rearranging and hybridizing themselves in constant flux.

Again, at this point Hofmann could have shelved the whole thing, passing the substance over to his toxicology colleagues and getting back to his day job of synthesizing chemicals for circulatory problems. But he knew he was on to something. Here was a drug with immeasurable potential, powerfully active even in the most miniscule of doses (it is still recognised today as the most potent psychoactive substance known to science by an order of magnitude far beyond the next contender). But which field of science could possibly be interested in such a thing? The answer, clearly, was and is psychiatry.

Once he had convinced his seniors about the importance of his extraordinary discovery (self-experimenting as the only viable method of believing the chemical's fantastic properties), there followed several years of phase one investigation of the drug by staff at the Sandoz laboratories, testing it on animals to evaluate it's degree of toxicity and potential safety for human consumption. The Second World War delayed progress for a while until, eventually, in 1947 Hofmann's colleague Werner Stoll at the University of Zurich published the first academic description of the mental effects of LSD on humans.

The laboratory studies had concluded that despite the drug's intense mental effects LSD appeared to be largely physiologically inert, causing little more than mild fluctuations of the pulse and blood pressure, and a dilation of the pupils. It had little effect on laboratory animals apart from causing some mild restlessness. Of course, had those rats and mice been able to talk we would have heard a very different story (but then had they been able to talk we might have wondered what we too had taken). In conclusion, the drug was certainly not considered to be physiologically toxic. LSD was deemed perfectly safe for human consumption and the plan was made for its distribution to psychiatrists worldwide under the brand name *Delysid*.

LSD Comes to Blighty for the First Time

In 2007 British psychiatrist Dr Ronald Sandison described to me the academic climate in psychiatry during the early 1950s:

> It was immensely exciting. We were looking for a new world. It's hard now to recapture the excitement of those years. During the decade or so after the war we were talking about the new Elizabethan age; everything seemed possible.[8]

In 1952 Sandison, like almost everyone else outside of a single laboratory in Basel, had never heard of LSD. But he went on an international study tour of Switzerland that year and, while he was travelling around looking at different psychiatric institutions, he got the opportunity to visit the laboratories at Sandoz. Sandison was fascinated by Hofmann's research with LSD, and was surprised that none of the other members of his party showed much interest in the work of the Swiss chemist. He made a point of returning to Sandoz two months later, in November 1952, and this time he came away with 100 vials of Delysid, which was most likely the first time that LSD entered the UK. Hofmann was gladly giving out LSD to any respectable psychiatrist who thought they might be able to develop some useful research utilising the new compound.

Sandison immediately began using LSD as part of his psychotherapy program at Powick Hospital in Gloucestershire. He gave the drug to patients who become stuck in traditional psychotherapy and soon collected a sizeable cases series for publication.

In 1954 he published an early paper describing a large group of LSD-assisted psychotherapy patients, 'The Therapeutic Value of Lysergic Acid Diethylamide in Mental Illness', in the British publication, *The Journal of Mental Science*, the forerunner of the *British Journal of Psychiatry*.[9] In it he described how using LSD he was able to re-awaken a therapeutic response from 36 patients who had become stuck with treatment resistance.

His managerial colleagues at Powick backed the research and in 1954 Sandison built a special purpose LSD clinic attached to the outside of the main old hospital building by a corridor. 'Of course it has all been demolished now', said Sandison in 2007. 'They kept the main building, but the very fine ballroom was demolished and luxury flats were built on the site'.

Just an Average Day at Work

Prior to starting the LSD work, all the patients had already been in traditional psychotherapy for varying periods of time; some for months or even years. There was no set rule but all of the patients had been failing to progress in normal psychotherapy.

There would be up to five patients for each session. A volunteer driver would bring them to the clinic at nine in the morning and the patients and clinical staff would all meet briefly. Then the patients would take their LSD dissolved in a glass of water. Generally, they would begin on a low dose, around 20mcg, which would be increased week on week until Sandison saw some progress. The average weekly maintenance dose was 150mcg. After taking the drug the patients would then retire to their rooms. There was a main corridor with the five individual session rooms extending off it. Here they would stay for the main part of the session. During the course of the next few hours, the nurses or medical registrars would go in and visit the patients as they lay on their beds. There was not someone with them at all times as many of the patients often preferred to be on their own. There was a record player available for them if they wanted to listen to music, and a blackboard for drawing on. Some patients brought teddy bears.

Then, at about 4pm, the patients got together for a 'wash up' group session to talk about the day's proceedings, before their drivers arrived and took them home. The LSD clinic staff had a very good working relationship with the drivers who played an important role. The patients got to know their drivers well during the course of their treatment because at the end of the day when they were still experiencing the effects of the LSD they would often chat to their driver on the way home. So the doctors and nurses tried very hard to make sure the patient got the same driver each time. Hence these volunteer car drivers became part of the therapeutic team.

Generally, patients had weekly sessions with LSD. Some had it twice a week. There was no set limit about how many sessions were offered, but generally if a patient had shown no response or progression after 20 sessions they might stop the treatment as by then it was assumed it probably wasn't going to work. Sandison did try using psilocybin with some of his patients at one point, which was also available from Sandoz. He recognized and appreciated that psilocybin had its place, as a shorter-acting and therefore slightly more clinically manageable alternative, but he generally used LSD as it was found it to be more effective.

Will LSD be the Next Big Thing in Psychiatry?

The staff at Powick were a very committed and involved team. The BBC made two films at the clinic: *The Magic Mushroom* in the 1950s and *The Beyond Within* a bit later. The psychiatric profession and the general public quickly began to take notice of this new experimental approach and a major LSD conference was held during part of the annual Conference of the American Psychiatric Association in 1955. Ronald Sandison was invited, and spoke about the work he had been doing at Powick. Aldous Huxley was also present, and he spoke about his own life-changing experience with mescaline two years earlier.

In 1959 Sandison introduced the term *psycholytic* ('mind-loosening') to describe the action of LSD, and in 1961 he organised a three-day symposium for the Medico-Psychological Association, the forerunner of the Royal College of Psychiatrists. A number of eminent psychiatrists, psychoanalysts, writers and commentators spoke at that event, including Tom Main and Ernst Gombrich, and all were very well received. Also at the conference was the British Member of Parliament Christopher Mahew, who, in 1960, had famously taken mescaline in front of a BBC film crew.[10]

This was all happening in an era before the popular knowledge and misuse of LSD. Drug abuse on a large scale was practically unheard of, and even within medicine there was no Committee of Safety in Medicines as there is now and little in the way of ethical boards. Evidence-based medicine was not recognized as a concept, and clinicians were effectively left to get on with whatever treatment they felt was right for their patients.

LSD as a Psychotomimetic

Sandison and UK psychiatry led the world in the early 1950s by developing the earliest centre for large-scale psychotherapeutic use of LSD. But his was not the first paper to describe LSD being given to psychiatric patients. That accolade is credited to psychiatrists in 1949 at the Boston Psychopathic Hospital (now the Massachusetts Mental Health Center) in the States, where, from the beginning, LSD's main role was thought to be not as an adjunct to psychotherapy, but as a tool to mimic and model psychoses; it was for doctors and other clinicians to take in order to glimpse what it feels like to have schizophrenia. The remarkable psychological qualities of LSD, coupled with the fact that it was a known organic agent with a demonstrable (though at the time poorly understood) mode of action, excited many researchers that here was a way of understanding how schizophrenia works at the brain level.

Theories were put forward, many involving the possible role for adrenaline or noradrenaline (epinephrine or norepinephrine), which excited interested researchers at the Boston Psychopathic Hospital at the time, not least because they supported the prevailing opinion of one of their contemporaries, Dr. Daniel H. Funkenstein, who had proposed a pituitary-driven physiological explanation for the modulation of mental states.

In 1950, in a study far more in common with the European development of psycholytic psychotherapy, Anthony Busch and Warren Johnson of St. Louis, Missouri, USA, published the results of a small case series describing the effects of LSD when given at low doses (maximum 40mcg) to 29 patients, mainly with paranoid schizophrenia or mania.[11] They concluded that the drug appeared to safely allow for improved access to their otherwise inaccessible mental states and proposed further studies to consider whether the drug had a role in enhancing psychotherapy.

Enter Dr. Humphrey Osmond

The suggestion that LSD could be used as a psychotomimetic, and that the psychedelic state could teach us something about the natural process of schizophrenia, prevailed in the USA and particularly caught the attention of Humphrey Osmond, a British psychiatrist based in Canada. Working at the Weyburn Mental Hospital in Saskatchewan with his friend and colleague, Dr John Smythies, he further proposed links between the mescaline state and schizophrenia. Smythies and Osmond published a small essay on these matters in 1952, 'A New Approach to Schizophrenia',[12] and introduced the Adrenochrone Hypothesis for schizophrenia, which suggests that adrenaline undergoes a degradation process in the brain and becomes a psychoactive compound, adrenochrone, which was known to have a low potency psychedelic effect and therefore explain the symptoms of schizophrenia. Osmond went on to conduct a number of important psychedelic drug trials in Canada throughout the 1950s in collaboration with Abram Hoffer. He gained particular attention for his work with LSD and patients with alcohol dependency syndrome.

Using LSD to Treat Alcohol Dependency

It is well known, both back then and today, that for a significant proportion of alcohol dependent patients when they 'hit rock bottom' and experience the terrifying effects of the Delirium Tremens (DTs) this leads to spontaneous sobriety. For around 15% of patients the DTs, a profound organic psychosis brought on when heavy dependent drinkers undergo a rapid withdrawal from alcohol, prompts an immediate and intense distaste of alcohol.

From their interest in mescaline, Osmond and his colleagues in the 1950s in Saskatchewan knew of the experimental compound LSD, which was being shipped around the world free of charge from Hofmann's laboratory to any psychiatrists who thought they might be able to do something useful with it. The product information for Delysid said on the bottle it produces a physiologically safe organic psychosis. So Osmond's theory was that, as the DTs is a severe and dangerous psychosis that can lead to sobriety, why don't we give our alcoholic patients this new drug LSD and see what happens? The hope was that the LSD would scare the willies out of the patients but with none of the physiological risks of the real DTs. It might just work.

So they gave their patients LSD. But much to their surprise it did not frighten them out of their wits in quite the way the researchers had imagined. On the contrary, many of the patients quite enjoyed the experience, but crucially it did lead to abstinence from alcohol. Osmond and colleagues fine-tuned the process further, adding elements of supportive psychotherapy and, before long, were able to boast of abstinence rates of 50–90%, which far surpasses all other treatments for the condition before or since. So impressed was the Saskatchewan Bureau on Alcoholism that in 1962 it went as far as to report that 'such excellent results have been noted by the bureau staff in individual cases, usually with resistance to other forms of therapy, that LSD treatment, which was originally regarded by the bureau as experimental, became a standard form of treatment to be used where indicated'.

There have been notable critics of the Saskatchewan experiments, with some people stating that the team did not use adequate controls. And some researchers — particularly Ludwig in 1970 — set out to rubbish the experiments by repeating them but with no attention paid to set and setting (which really *did* frighten the patients), unsurprisingly yielding poor results.[13] Nevertheless, the topic of using psychedelic drugs as treatments for addiction has remained hot ever since.

There seems to be a lot of sense in the idea that once a person has experienced a reaction as intense as a high-dose LSD session (Osmond was using mega doses), other drugs such as alcohol, cocaine and heroin seem rather paltry by comparison. This leads to cracks appearing in the hold of addition, which can then be further widened by focused psychotherapy. This was also the rationale behind Evgeny Krupitsky's work in 1990s Russia, using ketamine-assisted psychotherapy to treat addictions[14] — a topic we will cover later.

A notable further word in the Humphrey Osmond story is that of his relationship with Bill Wilson, who had formed Alcoholics Anonymous (AA) in the 1930s, and took LSD under Osmond's auspices in the 1950s. AA applies an essentially spiritual model of treatment through which to attain and maintain sobriety. In this context, Wilson could see the potential role LSD could play, saying:

> It is a generally acknowledged fact in spiritual development that ego reduction makes the influx of God's grace possible. If, therefore, under LSD we can have a temporary reduction, so that we can better see what we are and where we are going — well, that might be of some help. The goal might become clearer. So I consider LSD to be of some value to some people, and practically no damage to anyone.[15]

But, funnily enough, Wilson's support for LSD in the 1950s is rarely mentioned to the two million AA members today, and nor does it figure in the organisation's famous 12-Steps method. However, watch this space to see how the field of addictions — an area of psychiatry fraught with ineffective treatments and high remittance rates — might be transformed by the development of new research into psychedelic drugs.

Enter Aldous Huxley

The final mention of Osmond has to be to report on his famous meeting with Aldous Huxley, perhaps one of the most famous and noteworthy historical episodes of all, as it not only led to the writing of the one of the most celebrated popular texts on the subject, but also generated the very word that appears in this book's title.

Aldous Huxley was already in his sixties when he wrote to Humphrey Osmond in 1953 having been intrigued by one of the British psychiatrist's papers on the effects of mescaline. Huxley was a lifelong writer and lover of all things mystical. He was known internationally for his highly intellectual novels and essays, which covered all aspects of the arts, history, philosophy, human lives and relationships. He had explored in detail the religions of the East and was fascinated by the subject of mystics and altered states of consciousness, although he had never actually experienced these firsthand. By the 1950s, he was living in Hollywood, where the sunlight suited his poor eyesight better than his native Oxford, and he invited Osmond over to chat, but with an ulterior motive. He expressed a keen desire to take mescaline.

On a bright morning on May 4, 1953, Osmond nervously handed Huxley a glass of water in which was famously dissolved 'four tenths of a gram of mescaline'. Huxley was excited about the event, having effectively waited his whole life to glimpse the realms about which he had been writing for decades. Osmond remarked later just how anxious he had been about the situation, concerned that he would be forever remembered in history as 'the man who drove Aldous Huxley mad'. He need not have worried. Huxley loved the experience, and went on to write one of the most widely read texts on the subject, *The Doors of Perception*[16], which takes its name from William Blake's observation that:

> If the doors of perception were cleansed
> Everything will appear to man as it is, infinite.

Sharing British roots, both men were academics living abroad and both keen writers. The relationship between Huxley and Osmond grew, and a series of letters passed between them in which they discussed all aspects of this curious group of chemical compounds, the hallucinogens. Among other things, they pondered what these drugs should be called. Neither was comfortable with the emerging suggestion of 'psychotomimetic', as they felt the effects of these drugs went far beyond that of simply mimicking psychosis — after all, there were all the aspects of the undeniable spiritual experience that needed to be accounted for in a name.

Huxley suggested *phanerothyme*, which means 'to make the soul visible' and wrote to Osmond illustrating his proposed name with a brief poem:

To make this trivial world sublime
Take half a gramme of phanerothyme.

This suggestion led to Osmond's now famous reply, thus concluding the issue and creating an entire culture:

To fathom hell or soar angelic Just take a pinch of psychedelic.

Thus the term *psychedelic*, which means literally 'mind manifesting' was born, and Osmond first used it publicly at a meeting of the New York Academy of Sciences in 1957.

A Brief Mention of Al Hubbard

Huxley spent the last ten years of his life deeply ensconced in the then tiny and exclusive psychedelic culture. In 1955 he tried LSD that was given to him by Al Hubbard — a mysterious and shady character from LSD history.[17] An entrepreneurial shape-shifter, Hubbard is reported to have worked both within and outside official government departments, been a scientific director of the Uranium Corporation of Vancouver, and owned his own fleet of aircraft, a 100-foot yacht, and a Canadian island. He also travelled around the world propagating LSD along the way.

Huxley the Conservative

Aldous Huxley wrote several other works relating to his experiences with psychedelic drugs and his last novel, *Island* (which was the antithesis of *Brave New World*, his most famous book written years earlier in 1932), tackles the issue of the role psychedelic drugs could play as part of coming to terms with death in a utopian world.[18] Given the popularity of *The Doors of Perception*, Huxley can be credited as one of the first people to effect a crossover of the drugs from the exclusive world of the scientists into popular culture. This is ironic, as Huxley himself held rather conservative views about how the drugs ought to be used. He did not imagine that these drugs ought to be taken by the masses (as was the role for *soma* in *Brave New World*), but that they should, rather, remain within the realms of intellectuals, writers and artists like himself. In fact, he was a very reluctant figurehead of the emerging psychedelic movement, who crowned him as their leader in the wake of his little essay on his mescaline experience.

Huxley died of laryngeal cancer on November 22nd 1963, the same day as President Kennedy was assassinated — most likely a fortuitous event as far as Huxley would have been concerned, as it nicely overshadowed his own departure. On his deathbed, he instructed his wife, Laura, to inject him with 100mcg of intramuscular LSD.[19] This she did, as the other occupants of the house watched in horror as the news of Kennedy's assignation came on the television. Huxley slipped peacefully into the white light of infinity, cradled by Laura, soaring on the molecule he had discovered so late in his life, a molecule that so perfectly celebrated the state of mystical bliss and enlightenment he had been searching for with all of his marvellously erudite books on the subject of the human experience of living and dying.

Stanislav Grof and the Perinatal Matrices

In continental Europe psychedelic research was taking off. Stanislav Grof began sitting in on LSD psychotherapy sessions as an observer as early as 1954 when he was a medical student. He had his first personal LSD experience after graduating from Charles University School of Medicine in Prague, Czechoslovakia in 1956. This first psychedelic experience occurred as part of an experimental study in which he was required to undergo an EEG measurement at the same time as being asked to lie beneath a powerful strobe light whose flashes were calibrated to tune in to his corresponding brain waves. Needless to say, the experience was life changing and resulted in a career studying non-ordinary states of consciousness.[20]

He moved to the States in 1967 to work at John Hopkins University, later holding a position at the Maryland Psychiatric Research Centre, and serving as scholar-in-residence at the Esalen Institute in Big Sur, California. Through a lifetime of work with psychedelic drug and non-drug induced non-ordinary states of consciousness, Grof has developed a highly systemised theory describing how early pre-natal and birth experiences can be re-experienced when in non-ordinary states of consciousness. He described a detailed 'cartography' or map of the inner space of consciousness and used these methods clinically with his patients to help them recognise how their very early infantile and foetal experiences continue to influence their lives.

This form of psychotherapy differed considerably from Sandison's psycholytic method, which used low to medium doses of LSD in repeated sessions. In contrast, Grof has often proposed using a single — or infrequent, such as monthly — high-dose session (up to 500 micrograms of LSD) followed by subsequent non-drug sessions in which the patient explored and integrated the massive outpouring of psychological material that occurred in the drug session.

He has carried out pioneering clinical work on the use of non-ordinary states of consciousness in the therapeutic management of easing anxiety associated with the experience of dying. Together with Joan Halifax he published his work with patients suffering mainly with cancer at the Maryland Psychiatric Research Center. Then, when LSD was banned in the late sixties and most research fizzled out, Grof in collaboration with his wife, Christina, developed a unique technique of breathing, involving hyperventilation, to induce the experience of a non-ordinary state of consciousness. His Holotropic Breathwork© method endures as a popular form of healing today and is used by many people around the world. Since 1994, Grof has been professor of psychology at the California Institute of Integral Studies in San Francisco. He remains one of the leading figures in contemporary transpersonal psychotherapy and psychedelic research.

Harvard University and Timothy Leary

No history of the roots of psychedelic research would be complete without the Timothy Leary story. This chapter is no exception, although much of Leary's story, because it strays from the subject of developments in the clinical aspects of LSD, best belongs in chapter five, Hippie Heydays. Leary, of course, would be proud to be remembered for straying away from the 'mainstream game', as he called it.[21]

Leary was a successful research psychologist by the time he got to Harvard in 1959, having previously written a well-received academic paper on the measurement of personality characteristics. He was interested in how the human personality could be dissected into its constituent parts according to a fairly rigid set of rules that govern personality traits. His design even gained the name of the Leary Circumplex or Leary Circle in which he described, 'a two-dimensional representation of personality organized around two major axes'.[22] His system found patterns in human personality traits and focused on how the interpersonal process could be used to diagnose mental disorders. However, his life was to take a sudden change in direction, when, in August 1960, on a visit to Cuernavaca in Mexico, he was given the opportunity to try the local Psilocybe mexicana mushrooms. A self-confessed hard-drinking Irishman, who, prior to Harvard, had been enrolled as a cadet at West Point Military Academy (before resigning following a court martial for a bout of drinking), Leary's experience of altered states of consciousness up to that point had not strayed beyond that of alcohol. On leaving the army, he studied psychology and then gained his Ph.D. at the University of California, Berkeley in 1950. But it was that day in 1960 by the pool in Mexico that was to change his life forever.

Leary Discovers the Divine Mushroom

Leary had decided to travel to Mexico inspired by a *Life* Magazine article by the amateur mycologist Gordon Wasson. After the experience, he was so convinced of the transformative powers of the magic mushroom to positively alter an individual's personality and life course that, on his return to Harvard, he decided to dedicate his research to this newly discovered focus of enquiry, namely, the psychedelic drugs. After the mushroom trip Leary commented:

I learned more about my brain and its possibilities in the five hours after taking these mushrooms than I had in the preceding fifteen years of studying and doing research in sychology.

He set up the Harvard Psilocybin Project with colleague Richard Alpert using a supply of synthetic psilocybin, those little yellow pills provided by Sandoz. Leary and Alpert (who later became Ram Dass) set about running experiments in which they gave psilocybin to 36 inmates at the local Concord Prison.[23] Combining the drug with guided psychotherapy, the experimenters hoped to demonstrate that psilocybin therapy could lower criminal recidivism rates, which they claimed to have reduced from 60% to 20% in their experimental group (these figures were challenged when MAPS' founder Rick Doblin reviewed the study data much later).[24]

Leary Graduates to LSD

In 1962 Leary graduated from psilocybin to LSD when dosed by British researcher Michael Hollingshead.[25] Another flamboyant figure from LSD folklore, Hollingshead is not only credited with introducing Leary to acid, but is also responsible for giving the drug to, among others, Paul McCartney, John Lennon, George Harrison, Charles Mingus, Maynard Ferguson, William S. Burroughs, Roman Polanski, Allen Ginsberg, Donovan, Keith Richards and Alan Watts — who applied the insights from their psychedelic experiences in their various trades.

When he turned up at Timothy Leary's place at Harvard in 1961, having been directed towards Leary by Aldous Huxley, Hollingshead had with him a now legendary supply of LSD in a mayonnaise jar, mixed into a sugary paste. Although he had just one gram of the then still legal drug, this was enough for five thousand 200 microgram hits. Famous for saying, 'Acid was a bundle of solutions looking for a problem', Hollingshead lived in Leary's house, taught at Harvard and participated in the Concord Prison Experiment.

Leary and Alpert soon expanded their project and set up an organisation called The International Federation for Internal Freedom (IFIF), and gave their psychedelics to a wide variety of people, including artists and writers. The scientific controls around the experiments gradually loosened and they encouraged the trippers to simply experience whatever arose, then describe it how it was. Their voyagers included Arthur Koestler, Neal Cassady and Jack Kerouac, amongst others, who dutifully recorded their impressions.

During the summer recesses from Harvard, Leary and Alpert set up The Zihuatanejo Project, which was an idea based on Huxley's utopian novel Island. Paying members of IFIF gathered at the beachfront Catalina Hotel in Zihuatanejo in Guerrero, Mexico, where with Leary, Richard Alpert and another Harvard researcher, Ralph Metzner, they took part in group LSD sessions. But soon the Mexican authorities became suspicious of the crazy Americans' all night sessions of love and music on the beach, and when the media started to report their 'LSD Paradise' Leary and colleagues were ejected from Mexico and returned to the USA on a specially charted jet. Leary returned to Harvard only to find he had been fired. The official reason for the loss of his job was given as absenteeism, that he had been in Mexico when he was meant to be teaching classes. But rumours were circulating with the Harvard authorities that he had given drugs to undergraduate students outside of his project. The truth is the authorities had been getting increasingly uncomfortable about the amount of attention Leary and his crew were attracting on campus. For his part, Leary was making no efforts to play down the anti-authority viewpoints that spontaneously emerged in the context of his repeated high-dose psychedelic drug use.[26]

Timothy Leary's proselytizing of psychedelics did not end there, of course, and his influence on the developing 1960s counterculture in America and beyond became legendary — a story we will pick up later in the book.

God in a Bottle

Before his departure from Harvard, Leary played his part in a very important research study, The Marsh Chapel Experiment, which has since gone down in history.[27] Also called 'the Good Friday Experiment', it was the Ph.D. project of Walter N. Pahnke, a student in theology at Harvard Divinity School. Leary was supervising Pahnke as part of the Harvard Psilocybin Project at the time. Pahnke was investigating whether psilocybin could induce a spiritual-type experience in religiously predisposed subjects. The study stands out in psychedelic history partly because of the elaborate surroundings (it was conducted on Good Friday, 1962, at Boston University's Marsh Chapel), partly because of Leary's connection, and partly because it was one of the most beautifully designed double-blind placebo controlled psychedelic studies of its day — one of the very few from that that period, in fact, with such a high degree of scientific robustness; most other psychedelic studies of the time produced mere anecdotal data by comparison. Rick Doblin of MAPS reviewed this crucial moment in psychedelic research history many years later, in 1991, when he revisited the original participants of the Good Friday Experiment. They described how the insights and spiritual awareness gained that day have stayed with them throughout their lives as Christian ministers.[28]

But another reason why the Marsh Chapel experiment became so talked about was because it sparked a controversial debate, which still rages today, about the extent to which a drug can reliably mimic or, indeed, *induce*, a genuine spiritual experience.

In order to study whether the drug had actually *created* a mystical experience, Pahnke used a structured set of criteria designed by W. T. Stace, which were agreed to accurately represent such an experience. Stace developed the scale for evaluation by conducting a review of multiple written examples of the characteristics of the (non-drug) mystical experience, identifying nine core criteria that were shared and essential to characterise a true mystical experience. These, which were translated by Bill Richards and Pahnke to directly describe the psychedelic experience, were:

1. Unity
2. Transcendence of space and time,
3. Deeply felt positive mood,
4. A sense of sacredness,
5. Objectivity and reality (*real* and *known*),
6. Paradoxicality (*empty* and *full, alive* and *dead, microscopic* and *macroscopic)* — '*both / and*'.
7. Alleged ineffability (the realization that words can't describe the experience),
8. Transiency (the experience is temporary)
9. Persisting positive changes in attitude and behaviour

In his experiment, Pahnke gave half the group (ten subjects) an active placebo, nicotinic acid, which produces a mild tingling stimulation to fool the subjects into thinking they may have had the active drug. The other ten people received a 30mg dose of psilocybin — a large dose by any standards. However, despite the efforts to blind the experiment in this way, it became obvious within half an hour who had had which drug: members of the psilocybin group were lounging around the pews of the church in awe at the booming voice of the minister delivering the sermon; the other group members were feeling somewhat short-changed. The participants, all of whom already had a strong Christian faith and were studying theology as part of a path towards becoming ministers, were later required to complete a battery of tests that measured the quality of their experience. The outcome was a success, with results very positively in favour of psilocybin inducing a mystical or spiritual experience. Nine out of ten of the psilocybin group fulfilled the criteria for having had a fully-fledged spiritual experience, compared to just one of the placebo group. Pahnke thus concluded:

> The results of our experiment would indicate that psilocybin is an important tool for the study of the mystical (transcendence, ecstasy, cosmic) state of consciousness. . . . This is a realm of human experience that is reproducible under suitable conditions and should not be rejected as outside the realm of serious scientific study. . . . Our data suggests that when a person existentially encounters basic values such as the meaning of his life (past, present, and future), deep and meaningful interpersonal relationships, and insight into the possibility of personal behavior change, can be therapeutic if approached and worked with in a sensitive and adequate way.

God in Bottle? Not Everyone's Cup of Tea

Pahnke's work and the ideas that sprang from it stimulated a lot of debate, not least from the likes of the ex-intelligence officer and Catholic academic R.C. Zaehner, who at the time was the Oxford University Spalding Professor of Eastern Religions and Ethics. Zaehner was not a fan of psychedelics, having previously experienced a 'bad trip' with mescaline, and he went out of his way to rubbish the insights many people at the time (including Huxley) were attributing to psychedelic drugs.[29] Zaehner's conservative views contrasted significantly with the more esoteric reports coming out of those who championed the psychedelic experience. He claimed that any mystical state other than those that are theistic or attached to an organised religion must be inherently amoral.

Zaehner was certainly not alone in wishing to rubbish the value of the psychedelic state and distance it from other 'more natural and proper' routes to godliness. In a pamphlet released in 1966 called *God in a Pill?*, Meher Baba, an Indian guru popular in the West at the time, was keen to discredit LSD's ability to induce a genuine spiritual state, claiming psychedelics were harmful for the user.[30]

However, this did little to curb the enthusiasm of the psychedelic researchers. Many other experiments besides Pahnke's investigated the potential role of psychedelics as agents to induce spiritual experiences. In their 1966 book *The Varieties of Psychedelic Experience*, Masters and Houston wrote that after ingesting LSD 96% of subjects had 'religious imagery'.[31] Similarly, in 1964 a study by Downing and Wygant found that 60% felt 'a greater trust in God'.[32] A further study by Walter Clark, published in 1974, claimed that, after taking LSD, 100% of his subjects 'felt a subjective experience of "being in the presence of God"'.[33]

Pahnke's influential study continues to inspire today. It was the subject of another famous study in modern times when, in 2006, Roland Griffiths at Johns Hopkins University recreated many aspects of the Marsh Chapel Experiment — a subject about which we will learn more of in a later chapter on contemporary psychedelic research.

Things Start to Change and Doctors Get Nervous

Sandison had a very different approach to LSD than researchers did in America. In the UK, there was never a lot of support for the hypothesis that LSD could be a psychotomimetic. The nature and quality of the experience was not considered to be at all like schizophrenia, mainly because of the thorny issue of insight. On LSD, you know you've taken a drug and you can be assured that in the space of a few hours the experienced will have subsided, been resolved, and you'll be back to normal. Needless to say, this is a radically different situation from someone who has a fixed delusional belief that will not go away. Consequently, few psychiatrists in Britain thought LSD helped them to understand schizophrenia. Sandison never liked the term *psychotomimetic*, which is why he coined the term *psycholytic*. And unlike Leary's approach in the States, self-experimentation in the UK was less prevalent amongst health professionals in the 1950s. Sandison himself took LSD only once:

> It was an enlightening and valuable experience. Some people showed more of an interest in self-experimentation, but not me. I mean, how far does one go with self-experimentation in psychiatry? Does one have ECT?[34]

By the late 1950s, there were some serious problems emerging; not from the medics use of the drug, but from the military. The role played in the development of psychedelic culture by government military agencies in America and Europe is undeniable and well documented. At the time, the CIA had a low profile — though now well known — project called MK-ULTRA, which involved agents slipping high doses of LSD to unsuspecting members of the public and then studying them through two-way mirrors as they interacted with stooges to see whether LSD could be developed as a truth drug for military purposes. Lots of horror stories have subsequently emerged that demonstrate that the sanctioned government agencies carrying out this kind of work used methods and produced casualties that far out-strip any of the complaints of unethical practice that could be rallied against the medical profession at the time.

But another, greater phenomenon threatening to undermine legitimate medical research was the rising popularity of recreational LSD use. By 1964 the mass use of psychedelics within mainstream culture was just beginning, but Sandison had already been running his LSD clinic for over twelve years and really wanted a rest. Conducting LSD sessions was a very time-consuming and draining experience. Also, by the early sixties Powick Hospital was beginning to change. It was moving towards a centre for community psychiatry, and the hospital directors were really beginning to push it in that direction. There was also the emerging dominance of new neuroleptic (antipsychotic) drugs to treat mental illness, which placed less emphasis on outpatient psychotherapy sessions. It was time to move on.

It is estimated that by 1964 over four million people in the USA had used LSD illegally outside of proper medical treatment centres, and this is when the causalities (which were few and far between when the drug was used under medical supervision) began to appear. Sandison was asked to advise as an expert witness to a high-profile murder trial in 1964 involving a man called Robert Lipman who apparently murdered a prostitute while under the influence of LSD. There was a lot of negative press surrounding the event, and more and more horror stories about the drug were emerging in the press. Many were erroneous, but this negative pub-licity undoubtedly scared off many fine doctors from entering the field.

A Good Thing Turned Sour, But Outcomes Remain Good

By the mid sixties, there was a general feeling among psychiatrists that they didn't want anything to do with LSD. Patients, too, were reluctant to undergo the therapy if they had heard negative reports. It all became very complicated. Of course, there were increasing ethical considerations and bodies forming to control and regulate the profession. In the UK, The Committee for Safety of Medicines was formed in 1966, which introduced many new regulatory procedures.

Nevertheless, by this stage there were already many other psychiatrists in the UK other than Sandison who had developed their own LSD psychotherapy ser-vices, all of which maintained good results when the drug was used under careful medical supervision. There were treatment facilities at Roffey Park, Surrey; Guys Hospital, London; Netley Hospital, Southampton; and Bromley Psychiatric Clinic. After Sandison's large-scale Powick LSD Clinic the next most prolific provider was The Marlborough Day Hospital in London, which conducted over six thousand LSD sessions and fifty psilocybin sessions on more than five hundred patients during the early 1960s. It had very good results, with no suicides, no serious suicide attempts and only four psychoses throughout this period.

Indeed, the evidence base and success of the early use of LSD when used within the clinical environment was very good. Europe's use of psycholytic psychotherapy (using small to moderate doses on a regular basis with patients who had become 'stuck' with traditional psychoanalytic psychotherapy) and the USA-based method, psychedelic psychotherapy (using a single high-dose session followed by many non-drug sessions in which to explore and integrate the material that emerged in the drug session), were used to treat a wide range of anxiety disorders.

The 'peak experience' qualities of psychedelic therapy were useful for treating alcohol addiction, and the mystical and reflective qualities of the psychedelic experience were shown to be useful for relieving pain and anxiety of end-stage cancer, as demonstrated by a series of very positive trials by the psychiatric Eric Kast at Chicago Medical School in 1964.[35] Kast demonstrated that even when LSD was given without any formal psychotherapy it produced dramatic and sustained analgesia that out-performed traditional opiate-based drugs. This phenomenon highlights an interesting mode of action of the classical psychedelic drugs that may be due to its effects on vasoconstriction, and we will return to this later on when we look at some contemporary research with classical psychedelics to treat cluster headaches.

Did Psychedelic Therapy Actually *Work* in the 1960s?

In the 1950s and 1960s, before LSD was banned, throughout the world tens of thousands of patients were treated with psychedelic or psycholytic therapy by the medical profession. When the use of LSD stayed within the medical context, before it became abused recreationally, the adverse results were low and success rates were generally good.[36] Over 2000 papers were published on LSD during that period and psychedelic therapy was truly considered the next big thing in psychiatry. Widespread popular use of the drug outside of the medical environment had yet to happen (certainly in the UK, though in the USA even by the mid sixties it's use had began to grow, especially on college campuses) and the treatments were legal and freely available to psychiatrists. None of the media scare stories about nightmarish casualties had appeared. Instead, those psychiatrists who were increasingly choosing this avenue of treatment for their patients were seeing results that were overwhelmingly positive, describing safe and effective therapeutic interventions.

Dr Nicholas Malleson, a member of the Royal College of Physicians and the Advisory Committee on Drug Dependence, carried out an important meta-analysis of psychedelic therapy in the UK at the end of the 1960s.[37] He reviewed 20 years of psychedelic therapy in the UK, which included the pooled results of 4303 patients over 50,000 psychedelic drug-assisted sessions (the majority of which used LSD, though some also included were studies using psilocybin and mescaline). On reviewing this vast meta-analysis, Malleson found there had been only *two* completed suicides and only 37 patients who had demonstrated a prolonged psychotic reaction lasting over 48 hours. Despite these isolated tragedies, these results are very positive, especially when one remembers that at this time, LSD Therapy would generally have only been recommended for the most treatment-resistant chronic cases— for those patients who had failed to progress with other more mainstream treatments of the time, as was the case for most experimental and innovative treatments, both then and now in medicine.

By today's standards, to give an example for comparison, if one looked at a random group of over 4000 severe psychiatric patients over time one would see a great many more than just two completed suicides. This observation further strengthens the agreed opinion at the time that LSD Therapy was both effective and safe when used in the context of the clinical environment, under appropriate medical supervision by carefully trained professionals using structured and controlled therapeutic paradigms. Malleson thus concluded:

> Treatment with LSD is not without acute adverse reactions, but given adequate psychiatric supervision and proper conditions for its administration, the incidence of such reactions is not great.

As the sixties wore on, it was not only larger hospitals that were developing LSD services, but also many small and private organisations who were not subjected to anything like the sorts of controls around clinical practice that one sees today. And in those private practices clustered around Harley Street and Wimpole Street in London there was one such doctor who became an enthusiastic advocate of psychedelic drug therapy. It was the Scottish psychiatrist Ronald David Laing.

The Anti-Psychiatry Psychiatrist with a Passion for LSD

R. D. Laing first took LSD in 1960 and was so smitten that, when asked what advice he would give for those wishing to become a psychoanalyst, he answered: 'Number One, read the works of Freud. Number two, undergo a personal analysis and number three, take LSD'.[38] He saw the drug as an essential tool to assist professionals in experiencing the inner world of the psychotic or neurotic patient, and also as a valuable therapeutic device for loosening the ego defences of highly strung patients.[39]

Laing spearheaded the anti-psychiatry movement, which influenced many of us deeply. Looking back now, with more than a decade of clinical psychiatry behind me, I see that many aspects of the anti-psychiatry movement of the 1960s bear little resemblance to our present system. Back in the sixties, there were still many institutions that had failed to move on since the days of those dreadful nineteenth-century asylums. Practices such as psycho-surgery and ECT without anaesthesia were mainstream treatments, and many patients were still confined in hospitals because of their 'moral weaknesses' — for example, homosexuality was considered a 'treatable mental disorder' until as late as the 1970s. Even Timothy Leary himself, who one might have assumed to be more broad-minded on the issue, was not shy of talking about how LSD could 'cure' homosexuals by 'turning them on to women'.[40] So Laing had a lot to complain about and what he did 50 years ago was essential and right for the time.

The profession needed to have its cobwebs shaken off. In 1965, he founded Kinglsey Hall in East London, an experiment in psychiatric communal living in which the boundaries between patients and doctors — who lived side by side — were blurred. Psychedelic drugs were an integral part of the community. Traditional concepts of diagnosis and treatment were absent. The guiding principle was that 'to break down is to break through'. A resident of Kingsley hall in 1968, Paul Zeal, now a psychotherapist in Taunton, told me how group LSD sessions helped the residents to learn that 'rules were for discovering'. He described Laing as a containing presence who was respected by all, even when dissent was actively encouraged as an important tool for self-discovery.[41]

Laing rose to celebrity status as a result of his work and had many celebrity patients from the London glitterati for LSD sessions that he conducted in their homes, including Sean Connery, where his standard fee was a bottle of fine Scotch whisky and a limousine home.

However, psychiatry today is very much different than it was back in the sixties. The system now is not in any way perfect, and there is always room for a good anti-authority stance in any institution, but today we have well established structures of external regulatory control, powerful and empowered patient groups, clear lines of accountability, ethics committees and all the other joys of clinical governance and health and safety that are found in the modern world. But from my own clinical experience, the reason much of Laing now seems dated is in his concept that psychosis is nothing more than unrecognised creativity, a position that seems somewhat romantic and unrealistic. The idea that we should 'free the schizophrenics' by flinging open the doors of our hospitals and giving them an easel and canvas to express themselves (with the hope that they will teach us something about the world) just does not cohere with so much of the personal experience of people with severe mental illness. Most people with schizophrenia and mania are *not* closet artists, any more than most artists have psychosis.

Having said that, a recent study by Simon Kyaga et al from Sweden on 300,000 patients with psychosis *did* see a link between creativity and severe mental disorder, which is a good thing, I suppose, depending on how one looks at it.[42] This is certainly a field worthy of more research, which could be informed by the psychedelic experience. In a later chapter, we concentrate on the close relationship between psychedelics and creativity.

Prohibition and Ecstasy

Before we finish this chapter, there are two more important pieces of history from the second great psychedelic era that need to be addressed: the change in the legal status of LSD and the emergence of ecstasy.

Despite the protestations of those therapists who were using it safely and effectively with their patients, by 1966 tens of millions of people had used the drug outside of the medical environment. Rather than listen to the views of many academic and spiritual leaders at the time, who proposed a system of control that would allow for the safe use of the drug, the authorities, in their wisdom, made

LSD illegal. Suffice to say, this legislation did nothing to curb LSD's recreational use — which continued to grow, alongside the illegal use of every other drug — but the move was very effective at halting practically all medical research. The doctors, unlike the unscrupulous hippies who had no qualms about taking a banned drug, simply couldn't associate themselves with such a red-hot product. Consequently, medical licenses to use LSD experimentally became harder to get and many interested psychiatrists simply moved on to other projects, namely, those new antipsychotics that the burgeoning pharmaceutical industry were now pushing with vigour. Psychedelic research ground to a halt, not because it wasn't safe or effective, but simply because of socio-political reasons, which, in my view, is terribly bad science and left a lot of patients who may have benefitted from its use wanting.

But the banning of LSD opened up a new development, one that may promise to *really* be the next big thing in psychiatry: ecstasy, or MDMA. But before we get onto that topic, we are going to explore whether psychedelic drugs could be responsible for the very emergence of humans in the first place. In order to do this we are going back about one-million years to some psychedelic cave-dwelling folk.

CHAPTER 4

The Prehistory and Ancient History of Hallucinogens

Contemplation of Navels

Today, the concept of spirituality, and even more so that of religion, exists, it seems, on a separate plane from that of science. Many people, such as religious fundamentalists, scientific materialists and atheists will say they subscribe entirely to one approach or the other, but for many others these subjects are grey areas. Whereas spirituality is supported by faith and immediate inner experience, science uses a system of experimentation and testable evidence to support its claims. For the most part, science is comprehensible and verifiable and those things we do not yet comprehend, such as the exact nature of the universe at its moment of conception, remain nothing more than a transient gap in our knowledge, which those clever chaps at the Large Hadron Collider at CERN in Geneva are soon to discover. The world disclosed by science suggests that everything is very ordered and efficient as we move inexorably towards a total complete understanding of all there is to know.

For the record, I am a deeply spiritual, irreligious and scientifically agnostic person. However, I believe there is little empirical evidence for consciousness existing outside the brain. My understanding of consciousness is therefore best explained by the epiphenomenonalist point of view, namely, that consciousness is a consequence of our highly complex brains, producing the illusion of this phenomenon we call consciousness and that without a human brain there to appreciate it no such thing would exist. While I realise this view separates me from many in the psychedelic community, for me Occam's Razor (the principle that one should choose the simplest, most obvious explanation) supports my understanding of consciousness. On the other hand, God — if there is such a thing — can, I believe, be known through the psychedelically-induced peak experience. And science — if there is such a thing (which might then mean there is no need for God), in the meantime — can tell us everything there is to know about the universe. I appreciate this viewpoint I hold is ambivalent — which is why I have such a love of both spirituality and science, and why I remain agnostic.

The trouble with our current level of understanding is that within the modern scientific worldview there is little room left for mystery and myth, and there is little to justify residing in ignorance or loafing around pontificating about the really important things in life, traditionally addressed by myth and religion, which I feel is somewhat sad. Making up stories and inventing untruths, such as 'there may be a dragon over that hill' or 'don't go in the forest because there are trolls in there that will eat you' are seen as childish or superstitious nonsense and dismissed by religious and scientific adults alike. And yet we know children can teach us a lot about how to live fulfilled and joyful lives.

There was a time — not so very long ago in the grand scheme of things — when these myths and mysteries really did occupy our thoughts. They were not merely stories and time-wasting fantasies; they were seen as being true, revealing something real about existence. Until modern science emerged after the sixteenth century, we needed these facts — dreamed up by wise and knowledgeable elders — to protect us, to explain the unpredictability in our environment, to fill the gaps in our knowledge about the irrepressible forces of nature that controlled the hapless lives of fragile communities. Myth, understood as primitive explanations of the workings of nature, was effectively the science of the day. But this is only one view of myth. Myths also reveal something that sciences misses; spirituality, connection to land, environment, the past; moral instruction perhaps, illumination to guide us through different life stages. In the ancient world, there was no dichotomy between science and spirituality; they were one and the same thing, because these categories were not distinguished. No one felt the need to invent spirituality. It didn't arise out of some intellectual need for a greater depth in our lives.

It was only once our knowledge of science developed in the sixteenth and seventeenth centuries that it overtook religion and spirituality, and created the separation. Cartesian philosophy was also foundational to this direction in thought. But why and how did spirituality arise in the first place? In the next section, I will attempt to tackle this question from my perspective as a medical scientist and armchair enthusiast.

Sitting Around and Coming Up with God

A good question to consider first is this: Is it an intrinsic part of our experience to look beyond the superficial aspects of life and strive for something more? To do so, to make that metaphysical leap of faith from a purely intellectual standpoint would, from a modern scientific perspective, seem to be such a wild and fanciful thing to do that it is almost inconceivable that it happened. Even the most intelligent and worldly-wise humans of their day, gathered together in a cave around a crackling fire, are unlikely to have 'invented' gods and goddesses. Such ideas can't possibly have arisen from an intellectual or logical beginning.

I am very fond of the works of Terence McKenna. His ideas are so 'out there' that one is forced to react to them, either for or against. Arising from his exploration of the internal and external landscape disclosed by high-dose psilocybin, he makes speculations delivered in a trademark American drawl. His ideas range from the most astute scientific points to the most ridiculous, fanciful dreams and he himself does not always make efforts to distinguish which is which. He prefers the reader or listener to sort the wheat from the chaff and make their own mind up.

One particularly interesting idea that has made McKenna well known, which, personally, I do not think is as crazy as it seems, is that psychedelic plants and fungi played a central role, *the* central role, in the development of humans as sentient, spiritual, socially complex animals, which led in turn to our increased survival rates, the evolution of intelligence and the development into what we are today.[1] In describing this below, I have expanded McKenna's idea a little by throwing in some observations about autism and language that I have made through my own clinical practice and knowledge about the effects of psychedelic drugs.

Portal For the Immortal

The reason Terence McKenna's idea resonates so well with his readers is that it appeals to scientists as well as spiritual believers. What he proposes — to loosely paraphrase — is that the essential catalyst that sparked the development of spirituality in early humans was a psychedelic mushroom. This suggestion makes sense because it attributes that miraculous leap of faith not to a group of cave dwellers using the powers of their intellectual functioning to invent God, but rather to the organic process of a spontaneous mental effect. We have already established that the psychedelic experience frequently causes intense sensations of cosmic oneness. Many experiments, both from the 1960s and more recently, have demonstrated that previously atheistic people, when given a psychedelic drug or undergoing a non-drug peak experience (induced by other techniques such as asceticism, fasting, breathing, rites of passage), may describe their experience as spiritual. So it would make sense that it was a non-ordinary state of consciousness that first opened these ancient human's eyes to the possibility of a spiritual dimension.

Of course, it starts getting complicated when one asks whether or not psychedelic drugs simply act like lenses that allow us to see a god that was always there, or whether they simply mangle our brains and make us think there is a god when there isn't. Regardless of one's answer to that question, as a neuroscientist I am more interested in the simple and well-established fact that when we put psychedelic drugs into our brains, at the very least, it *feels* as if a god is out there. To understand what is taking place here can teach us an awful lot about the actions of psychedelic drugs and the mechanism of function of our brains. We'd also probably we'd learn a thing or two about God at the same time.[2]

Back to the Cave People

McKenna backs up his proposition that mushrooms played a major part in the development of human consciousness with the evidence that something peculiar happened in our development around one-million years ago. We evolved from *homo erectus* into *homo sapiens* at a relatively fast pace. Prior to *erectus*, we had been *homo africanus* for around five-million years. The evolution from *africanus* to *erectus* was painfully slow, but once we became *erectus* we then very rapidly became *sapiens* within a mere million years, which is but an instant in evolutionary terms.

So what happened during that brief million years? An awful lot it seems. *Homo sapiens* is a considerably more advanced model than *erectus*, with some great new added features including opposing thumbs, bipedalism, binocular vision and a throwing arm. But above and beyond these useful skills, by the end of this period we had developed language and spirituality. In the blink of a hairy eye, we had advanced beyond mere primitive animals into a race of sentient, artistic, spirit-worshipping humans, with increasingly sophisticated social communities, complex relational ideas and all kinds of stories for our young about the creation of the world, the deeds of gods and goddesses, and cosmic oneness of which we are a part. As described in *2001: A Space Odyssey*, we had well and truly stepped through the portal for the immortal.

Mushrooms Gave Us Thought and Thinking Gave Us Language

With the advances in our ability to manipulate our environment, we evolved from simple cave-dwelling hunter-gatherers towards complex farmers and keepers of animals. Early *homo erectus* lived with and around their cattle, and where there are cattle there are cow pats and where there are cow pats there are . . . wait for it . . . mushrooms! These early humans would have been in the habit of eating everything they see around them, which would include the strange blue-staining toadstools growing out of the cow pats. What happened next was nothing short of the opening of their eyes — or, rather, as Carhart-Harris at Imperial University has established with his recent psilocybin neuroimaging experiments, a closing of the eyes and an opening to the depths of the inner world of mind.[3] These mushrooms, we can speculate, forced our cave-people to go within, while spontaneously inducing feelings of oceanic boundlessness and unity. The ancient humans, their sensibilities heightened by the mushrooms, had no choice but to ask themselves some very novel questions: What *is* going on? Is this it, or are we part of something bigger? Are those really just clouds up there or is there some bigger scheme at work?

It was but a short jump from there to the development of cave art, culture and stories. Furthermore, McKenna goes on to argue that, at low doses, psilocybin increases visual acuity, which gave the mushroom-eating hunters an advantage over those who hadn't eaten the mushroom, and led to further selection for mushroom eating. But even more important is that we developed language.

The subject of language development is vast and far beyond the scope of this book, but one popular and interesting theory, proposed by Steven Jay Gould, is that language initially developed not as a means of communication with others, but rather as a means to hold a personal dialogue with ourselves.[4] In order to understand the complexity of our expanding, increasingly sophisticated external world — and, perhaps the new world of spirituality revealed to us by mushroom experiences — we needed to be able to have a personal dialogue to make sense of our stream of consciousness, to help us to *think,* to understand different concepts and hold internal representations of objects. In other words, when we looked down and saw a piece of fruit we were holding in our hand and then we lifted that fruit into our mouths we began to recognise that this series of events could be strung together into a meaningful sequence, or sentence: desire-fruit-hand-lift-mouth-eat. According to this view, it was only at a later point in evolution that these internal *thoughts* became externalized speech and communication: 'I want to get some fruit and put it in my mouth.'

V. S. Ramachandran expands on Gould's concept in *The Tell-Tale Brain*[5] when addressing the subject of neurological evolutionary theory, though he fails to consider the role psychedelics might have played in the development of humankind.[6] He describes how the human ability of Theory of Mind (ToM) — the capacity to appreciate that other people have minds — allows one to see other people's point of view and, by extension, reflect upon *one's own* internal mental state. Such a unique skill, which appears to set us apart from other species of animals, has allowed us to advance beyond the slow pace of genetic evolution to develop more rapidly reproducible tools for transmitting information such as teaching. Freed from genetics as our only means of progress, we have since left all other species behind. And there are clear links between ToM, psychedelics and autism. Indeed, Dr. Alicia Danforth, a psychedelic researcher in the USA, and others at MAPS, are currently developing a study to explore whether drugs such as LSD and psilocybin that produce recognised expansions of one's boundaries beyond those of one's own fixed ego, or drugs such as MDMA that have known empathic-boosting effects, may have clinical value in the treatment of autism.

As a psychiatrist who has worked extensively with children with autism, I would echo that it feels intuitively right that the extraordinary mental states produced by these drugs could have therapeutic uses with this disorder. Autism is all about being trapped within one's own shrunken, asocial universe. A drug experience that opens up the individual to feel instinctively part of a greater whole could be a valuable tool. A few studies were done in the 1960s giving severely autistic children high doses of LSD, with some noteworthy results.[7] Children who were previously shut off from the outside world or mute became animated and verbal, and laughed and engaged with their carers for a few hours, before returning back to their internal worlds when he drugs wore off. Such studies, which by modern standards provide little more than anecdotal evidence of the drug's efficacy, are certainly worth revisiting with contemporary scientific methods. But can one even begin to imagine the ethical issues in proposing such a research study on children today? If Danforth is successful in her study with adults with autism, I may take steps to propose something similar for children, who more than anyone deserve a way out.

The Mushroom Cycle

So imagine the scenario: Once the cave-people have gathered their cattle around them, munched the toadstools, increased their visual acuity, and improved their hunting ability they can now also develop a method for sophisticated internal dialogue with themselves. They can fathom out what the universe is all about, now they have glimpsed the cosmic wonder given to them by the mushroom experience and this expanded internal conversation may used also as an external communication tool. And it seems that those who eat the mushrooms, in low doses, also show an increased interest in sexual activity, which further boosts their numbers. Higher doses of the mushrooms — which, we can speculate, they began to go out of their way to look for rather than just eat accidentally — were contributing to their development of language by providing them with even more novel ideas to think about and then talk about. ToM begins to appear. They have an understanding about themselves and that they exist. They can talk to other people about their thoughts, wants and desires because once they start sharing their internal thoughts it turns out that others have minds too. Bigger brains, more food, more sex, more ideas leads to more sophisticated communal groups. Language and ideas spread through teaching.

If the cave-people begin to notice that the mushrooms — which by now may have risen to a position of high status in the community — only grow at certain times of the year then life starts becoming even more cyclical and seasonal. It becomes a communal ceremonial event to consume the mushrooms. This would fit in well with their increasing knowledge about the year's seasons. Then imagine that really high doses begin. For a few months of the year, a few people, those with the appropriate genetic predisposition for channelling and communicating the mushroom's message, become held aloft as tribal leaders, soothsayers, holy people. (It is notable that, thanks to Roland Griffiths' work at Johns Hopkins University, we are now getting excitingly close to knowing in advance which of us have an increased genetic predisposition to experiencing spiritual thoughts on psilocybin and which of us don't.[8]) Now that the cave people are thinking in an increasingly cyclical and spiritual manner they are able to reflect upon past generations and this naturally leads to the development of myths, legends and stories. Cause and effect becomes the name of the game. The seasons change like they do because of the forces that we glimpse when we eat the special fruit — we know this to be true as we have seen and felt it. *There is something out there.* It's not just about chasing mammoths around. There is a god. The mushroom is the god. Terence McKenna is quite a guy.

A final word, for now, from McKenna, which ties in nicely with the cyclical nature of psychedelic mushrooms (and also appeals to me because of my love of brewing cider). McKenna and others have postulated that these ancient people preserved their psychedelic mushrooms by storing them in honey. In this way, the early humans could try to make their magic fruit last all year so they were not confined only to the winter months for their precious ecstatic opportunities to worship their gods. Storing mushrooms in honey is a fine way of preserving them and one technique (among many others) that some hallucinogenic fungi enthusiasts still employ today. The trouble is that if one leaves honey uneaten for too long it tends to ferment. And McKenna speculates (there is little empirical evidence for this) that storing mushrooms in honey accounts for the gradual loss of these ancient mushroom cultures and a development of an alcohol culture. He suggests that from time to time there might be years when the mushroom crop was low and few caps were gathered and stored. Then, when the communal psychedelic ceremonies came around, the revellers, we can imagine, would be consuming far more in the way of fermented honey than that of magic mushrooms. So, if this theory holds up, they didn't trip and speak to their gods like they intended, but what they did do is have a right royal knees up. Laughs, sex and drunken fights were enjoyed instead of the spiritual awakenings. The likely result, sad though it may seem, was that the people began to gradually *prefer* the easy drunkenness to the, far more challenging psychedelic experience. Over the generations, by this account, the mushrooms got lost altogether, except for a few chosen members of the community who continued the sacred tradition: the shamans. Meanwhile, alcohol became the community's drug of choice and more sophisticated methods of preparing fermented (non-psychedelic) fruits were developed.

So, according to McKenna's speculation, not only do we owe spirituality, consciousness, cognitive development and language to the mushrooms but they themselves were also responsible for the rise of their very nemesis, alcohol. I guess we could all drink mead to that, if it is to be believed.

The Birth of Religion

If one follows McKenna's speculative argument through, one might conclude that the great influence of psychedelic plants and fungi over human psycho-spiritual development gives rise to the birth of modern humans. There are cultures, for example the Mazatec Indians in Central America, where psychedelic plants and fungi became the heart and soul of social and religious life for the community. For the Mazatec the mushroom was revered as a sacramental tool.

The notion that religion develops as a direct consequence of the organic influence of psychedelic chemicals feels intuitively correct to many followers of McKenna — myself included. Just as other major evolutionary steps took place through the catalectic influence of some organic or physical intervention — such as lightning striking a tree leading to the discovery of fire or iron rich rocks falling into fires giving rise to the discovery of metal — the inadvertent, *non-intellectual* influence of accidental mushroom consumption growing into religion through the spontaneous catalytic inducement of spiritual thoughts resonates with me.

No one really knows how, when, where or why religion began. We rely on archaeological evidence to give us clues about how the earliest humans approached spirituality. But there is general acceptance from the scientific community that when ancient humans began to bury their dead this represents an emergence of sentient intelligence and ceremony — something one does not see with any other animals except the elephant, who famously bury its dead and even returns to the graves of long deceased relatives as an apparent form of pilgrimage.[9]

The emergence of complex burial rituals among early humans amounts to the beginning of symbolic representation of non-material beliefs. And some of the earliest rock art, that of the Middle Palaeolithic period, up to 300,000 years ago, involves geometric shapes carved into pieces of bone which may suggest that the artist was experiencing an altered state of consciousness, whether drug induced or arising spontaneously. Certainly, by the Upper Palaeolithic period (40,000 years ago), anthropomorphic images and those representing half-human and half-animal images appear, as in the many splendid paintings of this period unearthed in deep caves in

Lascaux, France, that suggest these early humans were the first people to believe in many gods whose very image was fused with that of nature. With this development, we enter the territory of shamanism.

Shamanism

This is another vast subject and one that underpins so much of what is understood about the origins of religion and the role played by psychedelic drugs. The fact that shamanism is still practiced today throughout the world by non-Western societies gives us clues that shamanistic practices go back a very long way. For those readers interested in shamans, look for Mircea Eliade, who is generally accepted to be the 'father of the study of modern shamanism', with his 1951 book *Shamanism: Archaic Techniques of Ecstasy*.[10] A notable critic of Eliade, and the supposed link between modern day shamanistic practices and those of the Palaeolithic humans, however, is the anthropologist Alice Kehoe, who criticises Eliade partly because he was a religious historian and not an anthropologist, and also for not backing up his claims of direct links between Palaeolithic religious practices and modern shamanism with appropriate field study data.[11]

Scholars agree, however, that the essential feature of shamanistic belief is that it is method of communication between the human and the spiritual world. And there is almost always an implied healing or medicinal purpose to the methods and practice. Shamans themselves were — and still are — considered skilled herbalists, botanists, anatomists and physicians, not to mention their role as psychiatrists and priests. They can be seen as messengers, carrying knowledge and information from one dimension of reality to the other, transcending time in both directions to provide for the health of their community.

An essential component of their practice is that of the use of altered states of consciousness and this may done using a number of different techniques. The healing or medical component is inherent in the technique, and the shaman — doctor, priest, psychiatrist — is often assumed to live *primarily* in the spirit or animal world, which is accessed by others through altering their state of consciousness in a ceremony directed by the shaman. For shamans, who *live* in the spirit world, the ceremonies can sometimes represent their opportunity to take a foray into the normal waking consciousness of everyday people.[12]

Consciousness is altered through the use of trance-like drumming, dancing, chanting, and songs sung by the shaman of personal and group significance for the prospective spiritual travellers. The experience usually takes place at night. It is usually a group experience for the many members of the tribe, which makes it cohesive and empowering for the community, not just for an individual.

Sacred plants are an essential tool for altering consciousness. In this context, they are referred to as entheogens, which translates roughly from the Greek as 'that which creates the God from within'. There is very robust anthropological evidence for hosts of plants and fungi being used in a shamanistic context for at least 5000 years — basically since written records began. The links back to prehistoric religion may be more tenuous because, without any written records, no one can be sure what took place before 5000 years ago. But it seems unlikely that entheogenic use only started at the same time as records began. One way or the other, religions are very recent; the vast majority of the human spiritual lifetime has been lived for hundreds of thousands of years prior to the emergence of organized religions. If we can accept there is evidence for the role of psychedelic drugs in modern religions, it is a fair assumption to imagine that psychedelic drugs had an *even greater* role in spiritual practices during pre-written historical times.

Put plainly, despite the relatively very recent influence of Christianity's attempt to eradicate psychedelic spirituality — whether at the hands of the conquistadors or the Republicans — it really has never gone away and entheogenic spirituality still plays a part in today's multi-faith secular society.[13]

Many Religions Can Trace Their Roots to Psychedelic Drugs

Although contemporary organised religions have clearly contributed much to modern life and modern culture, including communal living — indeed, such religions might have served an evolutionary purpose itself — their autocratic structures are a far departure from the individualised experiential aspects of the psychedelic experience., When, on imbibing a fungus, one believes with all one's heart that the universe is good and that possessions, hierarchies and ego boundaries are meaningless it is difficult to subscribe to the autocratic dogma of most organized religions. But the roots of the role psychedelics have played in our spiritual development are not lost altogether and can be traced back with good evidence to several examples of recent human history. Some of these are discussed below.

Soma

This was a psychedelic drink taken in a ritual manner by the early Indo-Iranians, the descendants of the Proto-Indo-Europeans known as the Andronovo culture.[14] Helped by their invention of the chariot, they spread throughout Asia from the area stretching from Hungary to Mongolia around 5000 years ago. *Soma* is first mentioned in the Sanskrit texts that form the basis of the Hindu and Zoroastrian traditions. Of the 1200 texts of the Hindu Rig Vedas, over a 100 describe the mystery substance *soma*, which, when consumed, allowed for direct communication with the gods. The Rig Veda describes *soma* simply as 'God for Gods', suggesting it carried the highest accolade of all. There are lots of clues hidden in the Rig Vedas that suggest the substance was psychedelic. Many passages describe the visions and magic to be gained by drinking *soma*, the manner in which it transports one to be with the gods and become immortal.

> Like a stag, come here to drink!
> Drink Soma as much as you like.
> Pissing it out day by day, O generous one,
> You have assumed your most mighty force.
> (*The Rig-Veda* 4.10)

We have drunk Soma and become immortal;
We have attained the light, the Gods discovered.
Now what may foeman's malice do to harm us?
What, O Immortal, mortal man's deception?
(*The Rig-Veda*)

Or, if there were still any doubters about *soma* producing a psychedelic experience, this next verse should be conclusive:

I have tasted the sweet drink of life,
Knowing that it inspires good thoughts and joyous expansiveness to the extreme,
That all the gods and mortals seek it together, calling it honey.
When you penetrate inside, you will know no limits . . .
We have drunk the Soma; we have become immortal; we have gone to the light;
We have found the gods . . .
The glorious drops that I have drunk set me free in wide space . . .
Inflame me like a fire kindled by friction; make us see far; make us richer, better.
For when I am intoxicated with you, Soma, I think myself rich.
(*The Rig-Veda*)

No one knows for certain what the exact ingredients of *soma* were, but there are many substances pressing their claims. Some scholars suggest it is ephedra, others, notably R. Gordon Wasson, suggest it was the hallucinogenic mushroom *amanita muscaria* (fly agaric) which, when urinated, retains its psychedelic qualities, a fact supported by the Rig Vedas mention of 'pissing'. The *psilocybe cubensis* mushroom, cannabis and opium have also all been considered potential candidates as key ingredients of *soma* at one time or another. The jury remains out as to what soma actually was.

Eleusinian Rites

In ancient Greece, there was a 2000-year-old practice of worshipping the goddesses Demeter and Persephone, called the Eleusinian Mystery Rites.[15] The ceremony occurred annually and was part of a major festival, but the rites themselves were shrouded in secrecy — at pain of death — so very little in the way of written information is known about what took place.

The known details suggest that the ceremony began with a procession, followed by a day of fasting and then the initiates drank a special brew made with barley called the *kykeon*, before entering a great hall called the *Telestrion*, which held 1000 participants. Here, revealed unto them, were mysterious visions, including knowledge about how to attain life after death. There then followed a great party with feasting and entertainments, including a bull sacrifice.

There are, as with the Vedic *soma*, a number of potential pharmacological candidates to explain the apparent psychedelic effects of the *kykeon*. Suggestions have included opium, the *amanita muscaria* mushroom again (this mushroom gets around, cropping up everywhere in psychedelic folklore, no doubt because of it's classically magic appearance: bright red with white spots) and various other types of psilocybin mushrooms. But most attention recently has been turned upon the known fact that 'barley' was used to make the *kykeon*. This may have actually been dallis grass *(paspalum dilatatum),* which is known to readily become impregnated with *claviceps paspali,* a form of ergot, which contains high concentration of ergotamine, which can be used to synthesise lysergic acid — a precursor for the synthesis of LSD.

I saw an excellent paper on the subject delivered by the author Carl Ruck on the occasion of the 2006 conference in Basel to celebrate Albert Hofmann's 100th birthday. Ruck postulates that it is possible to recreate the conditions of the preparation of the *kykeon*.[16] Mixing together barley water and mint (readily available ingredients to the ancient Greeks), impregnated with ash to provide the appropriate alkalinity to power partial hydrolysis, the *kykeon* could potentially become a powerful brew. Whatever it contained, the result seems very much as if a psychedelic experience was at the heart of ancient Greek culture. The Eleusinian Rites were greatly respected for a long time. The ceremony itself was held with very high regard by the Greeks, and a great deal of attention was paid to inducing a non-ordinary state of consciousness to augment the effects of the psychoactive drug.

During the secret ceremony initiates — who reportedly included Plato and Cicero — described their experience of 'seeing and communicating with the Goddess herself': 'Trembling, vertigo, cold sweat, and then a sight, a sense of awe and wonder at a   brilliance that caused a profound silence'.[17] It certainly seems, then, as if there were something very profound going on for such a ceremony endure for such a long period of time. And, as mentioned, this example of psychedelics at the heart of ancient human culture may owe much to a considerably earlier use of the drugs in a shamanistic setting.

Psychedelic Drugs at the Heart of Christianity

Going into a church today one is bombarded with devices and tricks to evoke a spiritual mood and to honour God. Such devices also have the effect of mildly altering one's state of consciousness: the ethereal music, the coloured dim light coming through stained-glass windows, billowing incense, the assumed awe-inspiring mind-set is further induced by hushed voices and an obligatory reverence. All these features are merely quantitatively, not qualitatively, different from the psychedelic experience.

Yet the most prevalent view underpinning Christianity is that of chastity and sobriety, a rejection of intoxication with any substance other than alcohol as requirement on the pathway to God. Only shamans and witches adulterate their bodies with the devil's poisons. There is certainly no room for psychedelic mushrooms in the Christian way of life.

But, as with Hinduism, does Christianity actually have hallucinogenic roots? We have already noted that, by a very long way, the majority of human contact with the life of the spirit occurred as part of pre-historic, unwritten religions in which shamanistic rituals were the common form of worship directly linking the experience of humans to the natural world of plants and animals around them. And we know that psychoactive plants and fungi provide the perfect psychological cauldron, as it were, in which to experience such a connection with nature and the universe.

Perhaps Jesus was a shaman — a long-haired sandal-wearing magic medicine man with an intimate knowledge of the herbal and fungal botanic practices of the day, an influential mystical man whose stories have been distorted with equal measures of pious veneration and immoral bastardisation by those who wished to suppress shamanic culture.

Historically, there is certainly a good chance that psychedelic plants and fungi, had they been available to Jesus, would not have been subject to the same restrictions — both legal, societal and moral — that we associate with them today. Elaborate mushroom cults at the heart of Christianity have been proposed by some scholars and (unsurprisingly) rejected by the church. Of particular note is the theologian John Marco Allegro's 1970 book *The Scared Mushroom and the Cross*, which is well worth a read.[18] The Bible itself is full of psychedelic imagery, despite attempts to eradicate this in the many versions that have tried to tell the Old Testament and New Testament stories in retrospective recall.

Assuming the gospel accounts are factually accurate, what, we might wonder, exactly was the forbidden fruit that opened Adam's and Eve's eyes to see the world as it truly appears? Some have suggested it was the *stropharia cubensis* mushroom that grows in that part of the world, often at the base of trees. And were there psychedelic mushrooms growing in the Sinai desert when Jesus went to where the angels were waiting for him, and was overwhelmed by a kaleidoscopic display of colour? One may also wonder whether those shepherds were eating the fungal fruits of the meadows that night on the hill above Bethlehem when the shaman himself was born?

Another beautifully psychedelic description from the Old Testament is that of manna, which, when fed to the Israelites by Moses made them look toward the wilderness and behold the glory of Yahveh in a cloud. And the early morning gathering of manna is described in the book of Exodus thus:

> Then said the LORD unto Moses, Behold, I will rain bread from heaven for you; and the people shall go out and gather a certain rate every day, that I may prove them, whether they will walk in my law or not.

> And when the dew that lay was gone behold, upon the face of the wilderness there lay a small round thing, as small as the hoar frost on the ground.

> And when the children of Israel saw if, they said one to another It is manna: for they wist not what it was. And Moses said unto them, This is the bread which the Lord hath given you to eat.

(Exodus 16:14, King James Bible)

All the usual suspects of the field have given their support to the theory that manna is actually a psychedelic mushroom. Dan Merkur, in his book *The Mystery of Manna: The Psychedelic Sacrament of the* Bible, certainly seems to have found enough personal evidence to substantiate his claim, but as it stands there is not a lot of support from many other notable figures of learned theology.[19] I have to say, however, for anyone looking for liberty caps who has ever ventured out over the autumn fields of South West England at the crack of dawn amidst dripping fog, they will contest that this description of 'small round things' in the dew does not sound unlike a mushroom hunt.

Modern Spirituality in Europe: The Middle Ages and Witches

The Greeks were psychedelic users, and it was the ancient Romans that saw off the shaman Jesus. The Romans were themselves firm believers in whole hosts of gods and pagan deities, and were well-known to be rather partial to opium, cannabis and datura.

By the fourth century CE, the Romans had, of course, chosen Christianity as their primary religion and, in doing so, thereby ushered in the development of the modern world as we know it. And as we head into the Middle Ages in Europe we see Christianity running roughshod over everything in its path, sweeping away any remaining vestiges of belief in the ancient religions under the banner of witchcraft.

The links between witchcraft, mental illness and psychedelics are, to the hallucinogenically-trained eye, obvious. Ask any child for their classic images of a witch and one will be bombarded with the full regalia of psychedelic and shamanistic imagery: She lives alone in the wood, has an intimate knowledge of nature and collects herbs, roots, flowers and toadstools to make her magic spells, which she brews up as a bubbling potion in a cauldron that give her special powers such as the ability to fly on a broomstick, the ability to change her shape and to cast spells on others.

Psychoactive Plants Available to Europeans in the Middle Ages

While there is little historical evidence for the use of powerful psychedelic drugs such as psilocybin by Europeans in the Middle Ages, what follows is a summary of some of the plants that were used.

Deadly nightshade (belladonna), has been long known as a deadly poison. All parts of the plant contain high concentrations of the drug atropine, which causes a powerful anticholinergic reaction of blurred vision, dilated pupils and tachycardia. Used by ancient people as a poison, it can be lethal and still causes death for a significant number of people every year who mistakenly eat its berries. But when mixed with other ingredients and applied as a tincture, it also has a rich history as a medicine. Furthermore, as well as the deadly physical symptoms it causes on the way to death, the Belladonna intoxication also produces a dreamy state of delirium and powerful hallucinations. This was a popular ingredient for European shamans in the Middle Ages.

Closely related to belladonna is the **datura** plant, a very powerful substance indeed. Other names for this substance include jimson weed, devil's apple and thorn apple. It is a woody-stalked, leafy herb, growing up to two metres high, which produces spiny seedpods and large trumpet-shaped flowers. The seeds and flowers are more potent than the leaves and roots. It is taken orally and contains the drugs scopolamine, atropine, and hyoscamine. The effects, which can include extreme confusion, disorientation and very realistic hallucinations, can last for many days. There are few positive descriptions of human consumption. It used to be associated with medieval European witchcraft as a 'flying ointment' and is still used today in India and Africa by shamans. Indeed, when I was in Northern India I met traveller in the ashram where I was staying who warned me off the local 'moon flowers', telling me that after eating datura she spent three weeks entwined in her mosquito net, believing herself to be part of some insane wedding dress scenario. Suffice to say I stuck to meditation.

Another favourite plant for European magic men and women was the **mandrake root**. Apart from being a fabulously psychedelic song from Deep Purple in 1968[20] (and much more in the way of psychedelic music later), it is also a fascinating plant whose roots not only contain high concentrations of hallucinogenic alkaloids, but are also rather cool because they are twisted into crazy humanoid shapes that make the root appear as if it is a little living person. Legend has it that the roots scream when pulled from the ground and there are heaps of legends and stories associated with this plant. It is well worth a look of you find it down the market. Just don't ever look one in the eye.

Another is **henbane**. This rather beautiful flower has been associated with datura, deadly nightshade and mandrake because it was historically combined with the others in order to produce anaesthesia. Henbane contains plant alkaloids similar to belladonna and, alongside producing hallucinations and delirium, can certainly be deadly.

Witches, Witchcraft, Ergotism and Witch-hunts

The concept of witchcraft, which is broad and includes many variations all over the world, incorporates some fundamental common defining features. The main feature is the magical (I would say psychedelic) nature of the witches' practices, but another is that witches are commonly maligned and oppressed. Witch-hunts were frequent and span a very long period of history in Europe between the fourteenth and eighteenth centuries. They were a systematic demonization of ancient pagan religions by a dominant and often paranoid Christian church, and the fact they were carried out over such a long period of history suggests that these non-Christian religions were very well established and difficult to eradicate..

But witch-hunts were much more than religious persecution; they were a direct form of sexism and of stigma against mental illness. They were also a clear attack by the (drunken) sober herd on the psychedelic-using oddball minority. In some cases, the so-called witches were intentionally practicing forms of shamanism that incorporated the use of entheogens. But in other cases it could be that individuals, and indeed whole communities, were inadvertently victims of mass psychedelic poisoning. Ergotism has been postulated as the cause of the famous Salem witch trials that occurred in 1652 in Salem, Massachusetts, in which a group of young girls fell into a terrifying state of paranoid delusion, confusion and hallucinations accompanied by vomiting and convulsions. They survived but were then accused of being witches. There ensued a mass hysteria fuelled by the fundamental Christian beliefs that underpinned the community and the girls were eventually put on trial and executed. But it didn't stop there. By the time the community mass hysteria was over, a further 20 locals had also been accused of witchcraft and met the death penalty. In 1976 an American writer Linda Caporael proposed that ergot poisoning might have been the cause of this phenomenon.[21]

Also called St. Anthony's fire, ergotism occurs when the ergot fungus grows on a number of different damp crops, especially dark rye, where its black nodules are less easily noticed. It was not just confined to the Middle Ages and cases may still occur. Indeed, there was a famous case as recently as 1951 when an entire French village was poisoned by bread made from flour poisoned with ergot.

Stigmatisation of Mental Illness

While ergot poisoning may explain some cases of witchcraft mistaken for madness, in other cases witches may have simply been old men and women who were mentally unwell. At university I studied psychology before I did medicine and on that course covered the concepts of misogyny, mental illness and stigmatisation as explanations for perceived witchcraft. Mentally ill people have always been maligned and rejected. They often drift towards loneliness and isolation. At best they can become increasingly ignored, often actively persecuted and, in the case of witches, hunted down and victimized simply because of their differentness. Thomas Szasz — who we all loved on our psychology degree course, not least for the healthy rejection of clinical medicine he instilled into our minds — likened witch hunts to stigma against mental illness. His book *The Myth of Mental Illness,* Michel Foucault's *Madness and Civilization* and Erving Goffman's *Asylums* are all important texts for anyone who might eventually become a psychiatrist, rightly attacking the fundamental flaws and potential pitfalls that anyone so arrogant as to declare themselves knowledgeable about *other people's* mental states may face in their coming careers.[22]

Hunting Down and Persecuting Psychedelic Users Has Not Gone Away

Today's 'War on Drugs', as it applies to the judicious users of hallucinogens, is our version of the Middle Age witch-hunts, albeit in a far less extreme form — although in some countries people can still be executed for drug trafficking. It is an example of an alcohol-supping consumerist, pharmacology-driven 'masculine' dominance over the peaceful 'feminine' earth movement. The War on Drugs has as much scientific validity as the Middle Ages' persecution of witches. Punishments are metered out arbitrarily according to the whims and fancies of the local authorities. Media driven mob rule takes control. Being seen to be tough on drugs by vilifying the local pot seller is a sure way of catching an easy headline.

The pot-selling 'witch' may be lucky and could be sent home by the police with as much as an ounce of hashish in his or her pocket (I have heard of such cases, in which a tolerant police officer turns a blind eye to a fellow smoker and sends him on his way with a nudge and a wink without even confiscating his stash), while at other times whole squads of detectives can descend on a person's house and haul him or her off to a custodial sentence for the merest crumb of hash down the back of the sofa — especially if he or she is wanted for some other heinous crime, such as having been identified on video taking part in a direct action anti-establishment protest. Of course, there are many issues to the fore here, but the links between the way drug laws can be applied and the arbitrary nature of the Middle Ages' witch-hunts are not lost on many people.

Further comparisons come when one sees how drug users today are often medicalised, pathologised and described as 'mad'. Their ways are different from the norm, which is the same as saying not as good as the norm. They are sometimes held up and humiliated to make the healthy non-users look good, and described by a political and medical model that rejects and, at best, pities the drug user. But the situation is even more complicated. This hunt has now transmogrified into something more interesting in that, back in the Middle Ages, the witches were themselves in a minority; they were the last vestiges of a pagan religion being swamped by a tide of Christianity, or they were lonely isolated rejects with mental illness. But now it is the majority within certain age groups who use drugs. Among today's youth, there are more who have used illegal drugs like cannabis and ecstasy than there are those who have not. So now we are in danger of a truly occult situation in which the hidden majority are persecuted by a political system they voted in but are too scared to vote out. Talk about Emperor's new clothes!

Spaghetti Monsters and Pot Head Pixies

As we shall see in the next chapter, there still remain many ways to appreciate gods and goddesses. And it is a brave person who dares suggest a particular way is any better than any other — which means, of course, there are billions of brave people in the world. Whether they were discovered very recently (in the last ten thousand years) or earlier, it could be argued that each religious belief system is an equally valid tool with which to experience the spiritual realm — no matter how fanciful it seems. And clearly it is very easy to intellectually challenge religious beliefs. In 2005 a man called Bobby Henderson was so incensed that Creationism might be taught in American schools that he came up with the idea of the Flying Spaghetti Monster, which is a god with a wonderful story about it's creation, existence and continued presence in our lives.[23] Henderson proposed that his 'Pastafarianism' had equal rights to be taught in schools alongside Creationism and evolutionary theory if school boards were so crazy to accept Intelligent Design in the first place. And another equally spectacular story is that of the Gong Mythology, with its detailed and colourful descriptions of Pot Head Pixies, as influenced by a psychedelic band with their hallucinogenic imaginations working in overdrive.[24]

Given these brilliant interpretations of our fragile minds' incessant need to dress up the complex yet horribly simple understandings of our existential meaning, psychedelic spirituality ends up standing out as a perfectly valid — if not crystal clear — explanation of What It's All About.

The Varieties of Religious and Psychedelic Experiences

The psychologist and pragmatist William James wrote *The Varieties of Religious Experience* in 1902.[25] His simple, no-nonsense description of the wonderful colourful versions of spiritual experience to be found throughout the world captures the imagination and logical persuasion of anyone who reads it. Masters and Houston subsequently borrowed the title of that book for their brilliant *The Varieties of Psychedelic Experience*, which approaches the apparently chaotic display of psychedelic experiences with a similarly erudite and exacting science.[26] Both books are a great read and the latter is, in my opinion, perhaps the best introductory text to psychedelic drugs available — compiled, as it is, with the greatest precision and charm from hundreds of psychedelic therapy sessions in the early 1960s.

Above all, these texts show us that there are many ways to be and to worship the Unknown. Not only are all these ways of worship as valid as one another, but they are also, very often, relatively reproducible. Similar mental states — and indeed spiritual experiences — seem to crop up again and again regardless of historical and geographical boundaries. The presumption, as far as I can see, is that there is an innate human psychological capacity for spiritual feelings and thought — and since our brains are pretty much the same as they have been for at least the last 100,000 years this would make sense.

Wrestling Bliss Off the Church

Language has provided us with some beautiful words used by various religions to describe both the spiritual and the inseparable psychedelic experience: *satori*, *unio mystica*, the *Tao*, *nirvana*, *fana*. And it seems that many words, such as *illuminating*, *transforming*, *bliss*, and *cosmic oneness* have been somewhat hijacked by religions. If one wants to use these words, one must head to the nearest church, mosque or synagogue to use them safely. There is little place for them in a scientific or traditional academic environment. If one dares utter them in front of a psychiatrist, for instance, one risks ending up being treated to the spoils of the pharmacological industry.

But these words are not *religious* words *per se*. They are everyday human psychological terms describing valid mental states. I believe we as psychiatrists need to wrestle these words away from the church and bring them into the clinic as valid mental states. Just as we use medical terms to describe the mental states of anger, lust, fear, love and agitation, so too can we use words like bliss and enlightenment. The concept of the spiritual emergency is long overdue in psychiatry, and psychedelics are the best placed tools to remind us of the validity of these mental spaces. For if we confine ourselves only to the normal waking state, we risk missing a whole new level of understanding about the brain and the universe. Psychedelics may be an essential tool in helping us understand this level of meaning in our lives and the lives of our patients.

Conclusion and Confusion about Collusion with the Delusion

So why are these fascinating drugs so misunderstood? Is it because they are associated with drug abuse? Or is it because of the erroneous belief that there are significant physical dangers involved with using them? Perhaps it is because the War on Drugs campaign has been so successful at labelling all illegal drugs as useless and not worth investigating. Or is it simply because people are actually scared of transpersonal realm itself?

In many non-Western cultures, psychedelics are used as viable tools to access the spiritual world, whereas most Westerners tend to lead 'religious lives' without ever personally experiencing a truly transforming or enlightening moment. There are many similarities between the psychedelic experience and the experience of religious or mystical transcendence. This has been so hotly debated in the 1960s and beyond that in this modern age of neuroimaging it has become an almost moot point.

As a neuroscientist, it does not really matter to me whether the experience is actually religious or not. The point is it *feels similar*. So what does this tell us about how the brain works? Can exploring these mental states be useful for the field of psychiatry and, crucially, can it have therapeutic value? This is something we will be investigating in the chapters to come. But next we are taking off our shoes and putting flowers in our hair for a trip back to the sixties.

CHAPTER 5

Hippie Heydays, Ravers and the Birth of Ecstasy

'Meet the Hippies'

Where did the hippies come from and where did they all go? The simple answers to these questions are that they have always been there and they haven't gone anywhere. There was merely a brief psychedelic flowering of recognition of their existence in the late 1960s and early 1970s, deftly sandwiched between the grim post-war years and the screaming rejection of all things corduroy with the birth of punk.

The first 'Summer of Love' took place in 1967 in the United States and is probably best encapsulated by the 'Human Be In' gathering held in Golden Gate Park off the Haight-Ashbury district of San Francisco. That timeless moment of white lightning-drenched epoch-shattering glory is generally considered to the symbolic point at which the hippie counterculture and psychedelia reached their peak in the United States. (And by *white lightning* I don't mean the popular English cider consumed by teenagers sitting on war memorials in rural towns, but rather the Owsley acid created especially for the occasion and scattered freely into the loved-up crowd San Franciscan crowd.)

But for those in the know, who had been at the psychedelic game for at least six years by 1967, the party by then was well and truly over. And, of course, by the time we reach Woodstock in 1969 — coming as it did after the bloodshed and riots of 1968 — the 'come-down' was in full swing. As Danny said in *Withnail and I,* referring to the last months of the sixties: 'The dream is over . . . they're selling hippie wigs in Woolworths, man.'[1]

In the UK, however, our best hippie years were yet to come, with the development of the tremendous Free Festival movement, the Peace Convoy, the traveller lifestyle and the Stonehenge festivals, which kept those flared loons flapping right through to the punk era and encouraged an entire team of undercover police officers to lie around in hedges with long-range binoculars surveying a remote cottage in Wales occupied by goat-loving chemists.

Who's Going to Take All the Credit — or the Blame?

No single person can take the credit for the movement of these psychedelic drugs away from the psychiatric clinic and into the mainstream consciousness. Rather, there were a number of simultaneously occurring threads operating independently, together with the groundswell of social changes linked to the end of World War Two. Some of these contributory factors will be discussed in this chapter. Or then again perhaps it was simply the alignment of the planets, the Age of Aquarius, or whatever other bit of dogma one chooses to follow. One way or another once Hofmann's cat had been let out of Pandora's box it was only a matter of time before the world turned on.

The Beat Generation

At the end of the Second World War, there were a lot of disillusioned men and women, young and old — some who had fought, some who had experienced the horror of war through their parents — who then met head-on the growing circus of post-war 1950s America in which shopping and entertainment were peddled to the masses as the perfect antidotes to the intrusive memories of recent violent conflict. The Beats were at the forefront of the beautifully slovenly protest to this homogenized bastardisation of aesthetics. A decade before the hippies did their thing, these bearded visionaries trudged barefoot through the streets of New York, San Francisco, Paris and Tangiers, hitched and rode boxcars writing poetry, listening to jazz, taking whatever consciousness-altering utopiant they could lay their hands on.

Allen Ginsberg first took LSD in 1959 at Stanford's Mental Research Institute, apparently as part of an experimental programme run by the revolutionary anthropologist Gregory Bateson. Good friends with the psychedelic crusader Al Hubbard, Bateson had been involved in developing systems theory but is better known to most psychiatrists as the brains behind the double-bind hypothesis of schizophrenia. Ginsberg was deeply enamoured by the astonishing higher trance state of consciousness given him by his LSD experience in which 'everything seemed to be permanent and transcendent and identical with the origin of the universe', and afterwards he famously wrote his poem 'Lysergic Acid'.[2]

Later, in 1960, while on a trip from New York visiting Tim Leary, Ginsberg was offered some of Leary's Sandoz psilocybin pills which the psychologist had at home as part of his then mushrooming psychology project. Ginsberg enjoyed an intense psychedelic experience and reportedly stripped naked, cavorted outside in the snow, and tried to use Leary's phone to tell Kennedy how great psilocybin is and how it could be used to unite the world's political leaders. Perhaps JFK took some notice.[3]

The Beats subject matter, for Corso, Kerouac, Ginsberg, Burroughs and Ferlinghetti, was the streets and the real people they encountered on their travels across America and beyond. They wrote as they thought, fuelled by Benzedrine and marijuana, with a stream of consciousness, a flowing of words that cared less about structural form and more about meaning and feeling. Their approach was an antithesis of the ludicrous addiction of the consumerist hell sprouting up and being mindlessly absorbed by the growing generation of middle-class Americans proud to settle into their TV-driven quest for ever higher standards of living. It was the Beats that provided the backdrop for the psychedelic revolution. They were the ones who drove the bus that the stoned kids were on. They rapped like embarrassing, but very *cool,* parents while a new generation of teenagers prepared themselves for a massive social revolution. But it was a revolution in need of a magic potion.

There appears to be a clear paper trail in which Humphrey Osmond in Canada (who started out with mescaline in the 1950s) tweaked Aldous Huxley's imagination, leading to *The Doors of Perception.* But it seems a different independent thread took R. Gordon Wasson into Mexico, which lead to his mushroom excursions and that highly influential *Life* magazine article, which subsequently stimulated Tim Leary's fancy and sent him, too, to Mexico. One way or another the stuff got out there.

The decision by Sandoz to try to recuperate research-and-development costs by titillating psychiatry with Delysid, available free of charge to anyone who asked politely, did a lot for worldwide distribution of Albert's potion. And the CIA certainly played its part by setting up MK-ULTRA, which frightened, disgusted and enthralled scientists, military people and unsuspecting members of the general public in equal measures while also very effectively disseminating LSD widely into the population. Some would say, indeed, that the US military did more to bring on the psychedelic revolution than Tim Leary. There are lots of conspiracy theories around this issue, but the best books on the topic of how LSD leaked from the laboratory to the college campuses and became a worldwide phenomenon are *Acid Dreams* by Lee and Shalin, *Storming Heaven* by Jay Stevens and *The Brotherhood of Eternal Love* by Stewart Tendler and David May.[4]

One Flew East, One Flew West and One Took LSD and Bought a School Bus

Scientific experiments on members of the public are a great way for the Men in Suits to let the public know they have got something good in their medicine cabinet. In 1959, Ken Kesey, an aspiring writer, needed the cash and agreed to take part in a series of tests on new drugs as part of the CIA's MK-ULTRA program at the Menlo park State Psychiatric Hospital where he was working at the time as a night porter. Week after week he was given a collection of different jabs and tabs and told to lie around and then report his findings. It certainly beat the usual drab surroundings — and especially when he took this little pill the white-coated experimenters called 'LSD-25'.

Kesey had access to the cabinet, smuggled out the experimental LSD and began having soirees in the La Honda area of California where he lived. In the early sixties the time was right, as he said later, to push the boundaries, to go down deeper in the oceans and up higher in the skies. The space race was in full swing, he was an artist on the edge of the Beat Generation and people everywhere were being encouraged to climb their way out of the PTSD-induced experience of the war, and to expand their cultural, societal and personal horizons. Besides, it was great fun.

Fun, riotous fun, was a central part of the subsequent Merry Pranksters group that emerged, forming around Kesey like a high, grinning cat. Kesey was growing in stature as an artist alongside the creative imaginations of the LSD he and his friends were using. It was while under the influence of LSD in 1959 that he wrote large sections of his book *One Flew Over the Cuckoo's Nest*, which was soon to become a massive bestseller and catapult him into the literary history books.[5] The story centres upon a broom-pushing psychiatric patient, the giant Native American, 'Chief', and describes the impassive agony of life in the mental institute, endlessly sweeping the spotless corridors. There are sections in Kesey's famous book (which never actually refers to LSD, yet is an undoubted psychedelic classic) in which there is a 'white cloud', described as 'the combine', the insidious controlling force that keeps all the hapless patients institutionalised. The cloud descends over everyone, blunts their minds and blurs the edges of acceptable familiarity, moulding the inhabitants of the hospital into a conglomerated mass of brainless automatons. This is a far cry from the joyous experience of taking a psychedelic drug in sundrenched hippie meadows that was yet to come later in the decade. Instead, it is a reliable description of what happens when no attention is paid to the set and setting, and the internal worlds are left to run with abandon in a frightening environment like an authoritarian mental institution.

On the back of the success of his book, Kesey and his tribe of Merry Pranksters took off in 1964 on a legendary road trip in an old Harvester school bus painted in fabulous psychedelic regalia, driven by Neal Cassady, the larger-than-life Beat extraordinaire, friend of Jack Kerouac and the inspiration for the wonderful character Dean Moriarty in Kerouac's *On the Road*.[6] Cassady, high on amphetamine, came with the perfect credentials to carry the tripping crew at breakneck speeds through the unsuspecting innocent towns of middle America. The Pranksters mission was to cause havoc, to push boundaries and excite and shock people. It worked. Later these adventures were immortalized in Tom Wolfe's *The Electric Kool Aid Acid Test* — an absolute must-read for a wonderful description of this period of American history.[7]

The Californian Proto-Hippies Get a Place of Their Own

In 1962, on the impossibly beautiful coast in Big Sur, California, Michael Murphy and Dick Price brought the Esalen Institute to into existence. Its stunning 120-acre site, provided a perfect platform for the discussion and dissemination of humanistic and transpersonal ideas, as it still does today. All manner of Western and Eastern philosophical thinking from yoga to ecology and massage have been explored over the years, with residents staying amidst the serene landscape perched on the cliffs above the crashing waves of the Pacific coast south of San Francisco. Since it's inauguration, the likes of Aldous Huxley, Stanislav Grof, Allen Ginsberg,

Carlos Castaneda, Gregory Bateson, Deepak Chopra, Albert Hofmann, Richard Alpert, Rupert Sheldrake, Terence McKenna, John C. Lilly, Ken Kesey, Abraham Maslow, Fritz Perls, Carl Rogers, Alan Watts, Andrew Weil, Robert Anton Wilson and Joseph Campbell have all held workshops and talks at the institute; and Gary Snyder, Michael McClure, Lawrence Ferlinghetti, Allen Ginsberg, Kenneth Rexroth, and Robert Bly have held poetry readings there too. Naturally, such a place became a central stop for many on the psychedelic intellectual journey of the sixties, including for a lot of popular music stars of the day and since.[8]

Literally, Psychedelically Mind-expanding Words

In the 1960s, not only was the use of LSD as a recreational drug growing, but there was also a blossoming appreciation of the multicultural aspects of natural psychedelic drugs. People became interested in peyote, magic mushrooms and ayahuasca, and all the colourful culture that surrounds these practices.

Shamanism became a popular subject and people swallowed the whole caboodle of holistic change, embracing a new paradigm of thinking, alternative medicine and ecology as readily as they swallowed their acid. Literary works alluding to alternative lifestyles — from Alistair Crowley or the idealists of the 1920s Blooms-bury set — were embraced. LSD encouraged an escape from the city and a drift towards Mother Nature, an acceptance of seemingly archaic ideas about communal living and getting back to the land. Large sections of contemporary society had their eyes opened to the destruction of the environment, the modern green movement emerged, and previously decimated sections of the population — for example, the Native Americans — were embraced and protests about their mis-treatment by modern America grew.

Twentieth-century shamans wrote about their experiences and new awakenings. Carlos Castaneda's 1968 book *The Teachings of Don Juan* described a personal journey into contemporary shamanism and remains a student classic today.[9] Throughout the sixties and since, there has been a seemingly endless stream of books about the politics, science and art of the psychedelic experience, not to men-tion many people's accounts of their personal experiences using a whole host of drugs, some of which are tremendously interesting and some, which one can imag-ine, are mind-numbingly dull. I suppose you have to be there really.

Did JFK Drop LSD?

This question has been asked by a lot of people. The association between Kennedy and acid comes from a three-way friendship: Kennedy had a close relationship with the socialite painter Mary Eno Pinchot Meyer and she was also in a close relationship at the time with Tim Leary. Mary's friendship with the president was intimate, and, meanwhile, her regular visits to Leary in Harvard made sure that plenty of cannabis and LSD found its way into the Whitehouse during 1962 and 1963. Mary considered herself on a secret mission to propagate LSD to as many powerful members of the government as possible in order to spread the love and avoid nuclear war. In his memoirs from much later in life, Leary confessed that he felt Mary was at least partially successful in encouraging the president to take a few steps closer to nuclear disarmament because of the transformative influence of LSD. But we may never know the truth of what went on between Mary Eno Pinchot Meyer and Kennedy, as she was mysteriously murdered — a year after Kennedy — in 1964.[10]

Unless one is open to conspiracy theories, it is probably best not to speculate what might have been going on. That said, there is nothing especially conspiratorial to imagine Kennedy took LSD. After all, he was an intelligent, switched-on and highly perceptive person. It is certainly conceivable, especially given the anecdotal circumstantial evidence, that he might have experimented with what was one of the most important social and philosophical pastimes of the day.

Leary Leaves Harvard and the Fun Really Begins

Earlier, we left Tim Leary's story as he was given his marching orders from Harvard. Interested to see how creative people behaved under the influence of the drug, he set about giving LSD to as many people as possible outside the clinical environment. A number of important writers and musicians of the day were introduced to it's unique mental spaces during this period.

In 1963, Leary eventually found his spiritual home in the form a massive mansion set in over 100 acres of private countryside estate near the town of Millbrook in New York State. Lent to him by the millionaire Hitchcock family, this became *the* place to go and be part of the newly developing psychedelic scene. It was from here that Tim Leary, now having shed what fragile ties he might still have held to Harvard and the conventional world of the establishment since taking his first mushroom trip, allowed himself and his willing followers to enter into a beautiful, swirling maelstrom of colours and escapades that were new to them all. As the Jefferson Airplane said, 'I'm doing things that haven't got a name yet'.

Leary's mental development was going deeper than anyone thought imaginable, heading into the territory of a fully formed religious movement. His *League for Spiritual Development* (nice acronym) was shaping into a loosely structured method of attaining spiritual enlightenment through the use of LSD and other psychedelics. Perhaps because of, or in spite of, his grounding in clinical psychology, there was a great deal of method and purpose to Leary's work. In his spoken words and writings, he *always*, without exception, talked of the respect one must have for psychedelic drugs. He never described a gung-ho or frivolous approach. He was clear that caution and a judicious and reverent attitude were essential to their use. Although he was not as tightly restricted as Huxley (who suggested the psychedelics ought not be available to large numbers of the general public but only for appropriately highly-tuned academics and artists), Leary was a good distance from the Ken Kesey approach, whose prankster attitude was always, quite transparently, to go too far and get as freaked out as possible. For Kesey, life, after all, may be interpreted as but a joke — and few experiences are better at pointing this out than a high-dose psychedelic session.

Suddenly LSD is Everywhere

Nevertheless, both Kesey's madness and Leary's controlled approach provoked complete and total revulsion in the authorities, who were keen to hold on to their grip of consciousness-control. If people looked within too often, they realized, they forgot to look in the shopping malls and sign up at the military academies, and that simply wasn't good for business or for the country. But there was little they could do. LSD was fast becoming the next big thing on the US college campuses. By 1965 over two million people in the States had taken LSD outside of the clinical or military test environment. This was never supposed to happen! Consciousness-expanding LSD use coupled very neatly with left-wing protests, anti-authority sentiments and, above all, the arts. And an awful lot of this crystallization of expanded thinking was concentrating increasingly on the West and East coasts of America.

New York was a melting pot for the growing underground movement, always frequented by the Beats, together with a healthy folk and art scene clustered around the coffee shops of Greenwich Village. And San Francisco has always accepted the cultural waifs and strays of the planet. Since the 1940s, it had seen a drift of open-minded people congregating in the wooden housed hills over-looking that foggy bay, especially the Haight-Ashbury district. LSD was bound to flourish here.

The role of the Vietnam War in the development of the psychedelic scene is undeniable. What better antithesis could there be of the LSD experience than a brutal televised war that dragged teenagers kicking and screaming away from their music and dropped them into the dark jungle thousands of miles away from home? If it is an intrinsic and spontaneous characteristic of an LSD trip to feel the love, then people now had many more reasons to strive for it. Britain lacked such a war, which might explain in part the more nostalgic, gentle approach to psychedelia that we saw in the UK.

The Psychedelic Music Scene

The genre of music dedicated to psychedelia is very close to my heart.[11] There are lots of good books to read about Haight-Ashbury and the development of the psychedelic scene. One of my favourites, with lots of local information and stories of the bands from the area, is Charles Perry's *The Haight-Ashbury*.[12] There are a lot of potential contenders for 'the first psychedelic band' so I will not try and speculate who it might be. But one might imagine it is a safe bet to suggest they came from around the Bay Area. Or maybe not . . .

Around 1963, an unusual scene, centred on a strange cowboy-throwback establishment, The Red Dog Saloon in Virginia City, Nevada, was developing. Growing numbers of artists and musicians were gathering there, dressing in vintage threads, carrying guns and getting loaded on peyote as part of an experimental tribal family established by Chandler A. Laughlin III. By 1965, this had become the place to hang out if you were a band interested in taking LSD and other substances. People came to get loaded and get up close to nature and in touch with the historical roots of Native America. Among other bands that played the Red Dog Saloon included

Big Brother and the Holding Company, Jefferson Airplane, Quicksilver Messenger Service and The Charlatans — who, more than the others, are often credited as being the first *truly* psychedelic band.

By this time, if one were interested, one was no longer entirely reliant on the increasingly hard-to-find Swiss Sandoz LSD, but could rather get fuelled on the widely available sacrament being produced locally in vast quantities by the chemist Owsley Stanley III, who, in 1965, was living in Berkeley and flooding the San Francisco scene with his chemical product. It is arguable, then, that 1965 in San Francisco was where hippies and the public phase of non-medical psychedelia all began. And especially the music.

On his return to La Honda from his bus trip in 1964, Ken Kesey held frequent psychedelic parties in the woods at his house. These became the basis for the famous 'Acid Tests' in which he and the Pranksters colluded to create spectacular environments for people to try LSD for the first time. Visitors knew what to expect. The sign at the end of the lane that lead to his cabin in the woods had been modified to read 'No Left Turn Unstoned'. At this time the drug was not yet illegal and it was increasingly available for anyone interested in trying it. Many people were wishing to do so and they congregated for these parties, firstly in their dozens, then in the hundreds. Before long the Acid Tests were taken on the road, with happenings rolled-out throughout California, played to packed halls of thousands of saucer-eyed revellers, put on by Kesey and the Pranksters with their Day-Glo painted craziness and improvised sounds. Using banks of audio equipment and cameras they wired the place for sound and projected back to people their own wails of ecstasy and confusion live as they happened — everything designed to twist the senses and expand the boundaries of reality.

And there was no better soundtrack for this experience than a weirdly familiar traditional country-roots-jazz-rock improvisational jam band like The Warlocks, a bunch of kids from San Francisco who played extended instrumental sets under the influence of swirling dials and patterned sounds emanating from the speaker stacks. They were later to become The Grateful Dead and they had their first gig in 1965 at Ken Kesey's Acid Test in San Jose, California.

Read All About It

By 1966 the Haight-Ashbury hippie scene had its very own shop and newspaper. 'The Psychedelic Shop' on Haight Street, run by Ron and Jay Thelin, which became the place to go for candles, papers, comics, posters, clothes and all the other necessary paraphernalia for those looking to get involved, or just hang around and fossilize into the surroundings. The Thelin brothers subsequently put up cash to start the first underground newspaper, *The San Francisco Oracle*, which was edited by Allen Cohen and showcased the latest sounds and parties, and provided a place to read about the exploits of Ginsberg, Leary and the rest of the characters embodying/portraying alternative versions of American life. The paper was known for it's colourful psychedelic artwork, directed by Michael Bowen. From here psychedelia expanded exponentially.

Hundreds of bands were developing their peculiar brand of esoteric sounds. In Berkeley, a 'right on' student activist jug band, Country Joe and the Fish, were brewing up their own versions of electric music for the mind and body, spawning a brilliant album that could well hold the prize for being the first record entirely conceived, written, produced and performed on LSD ('In our quest to be the greatest psychedelic band we must have taken more acid than all the rest put together!', as Joe McDonald said).

Psychedelic music was clearly designed to both emulate the sensations of the acid experience and be enjoyed in a similar state of mind. All of this was converging on San Francisco and would lead eventually to the Bay Area's first major record-label signing for a psychedelic band, which was for The Jefferson Airplane with their *Surrealistic Pillow* album in 1966. Psychedelic music had well and truly arrived and it was all very West-coast California, but nevertheless, the most influential musical force at the time — and soon to be leading the genre of psychedelic music itself — was coming from the other side of the pond.

It's All Too Much

The album *Rubber Soul* was The Beatles' cannabis LP and marked the permanent loss of the mop-top clean image. Bob Dylan had introduced them to weed in 1964 and all those introspective, soul-searching mellow acoustic songs on *Rubber Soul* had pot all over them. But by the time *Revolver* came out in July 1966, they were increasingly experimenting with LSD — at least John, George and Ringo were — they had begun taking the sacrament shortly before the more cautious Paul. When the album ended with the splendidly psychedelic *Tomorrow Never Knows*, it was as if mainstream psychedelic music was here to stay. With its lyrics taken from Tim Leary's version of *The Tibetan Book of the Dead*, *The Psychedelic Experience*, the opening line 'Turn off your mind, relax and float downstream' and the backing track, were designed to be reminiscent of a thousand chanting monks; it was clear nothing would ever be the same again.

Despite what more hard-core psychedelic music fans might say, it is difficult to deny that The Beatles led the way musically throughout the sixties and their influence in psychedelic music was keenly felt. Admittedly, they weren't taking as much acid and were not anything like as involved in the psychedelic culture as the San Francisco bands, but pop artists everywhere looked to them for sonic inspiration, and their arrangements and instrumentation were copied everywhere.

In truth, so many bands fed off one another and The Byrds can link their roots back to Dylan just as The Beach Boys do to The Beatles, and The Beatles, in turn, themselves pay many tributes to The Byrds. In the final analysis, they all look back to Little Richard, Muddy Waters and Robert Johnson. But it was the production techniques and creativity of The Beatles that so many musicians picked up on, including psychedelic bands from coast to coast. *Sergeant Pepper's Lonely Hearts Club Band* was the album most obviously leaning towards the use of LSD, but, in fact, the albums *Magical Mystery Tour* and *Yellow Submarine* contain the most classically psychedelic songs. One way or another — and I'm no Beatles expert, though I guess there are one or two out there — once the lysergic bug had been caught, by 1967 it was catapulted everywhere, the concept of psychedelia spread worldwide and made everyone sit up and listen.

It is fair to say that almost every well-known pop band at the time made at least one album or single that leant towards the cosmic angle (even Cliff Richard went mildly weird on a couple of his 1968 singles) such was the mainstream appeal of psychedelia at the time. One simply *had* to wear flowers and scarves, burn incense and talk about the inner world — just as kids today wear . . . whatever kids today wear. The English approach was always slightly more whimsical and tongue in cheek than the serious mind-benders coming from the States — just as Ronald Sandison's gentle psycholytic therapy technique contrasts slightly with Leary and Grof's high-dose peak experience approach. Throughout the songs of The Beatles, The Small Faces, The Pretty Things, Traffic, Cream and even Hendrix's early stuff there is the very English sentiment that one can take a trip, stroll through heavenly gardens of delight then come down and be home for tea, clear-headed and ready to meet the wife. But the American approach was often considerably more mystical (Country Joe and The Fish, Love, JK and Co., HP Lovecraft, etc.) or just plain 'out there' sixties punk, as in the 13th Floor Elevators and The Seeds. Note that I quite transparently consider The Jimi Hendrix Experience here as an English band. The better part of their career and the band's management and record label all came from England. Sorry if that offends American readers keen to hold on to Jimi. He's ours! In return, you can keep one of our TV talent show winners.

Psychedelic music got heavier as the decade progressed towards Woodstock and Altamont, and then fell into the seventies in a screech of rock as artists began turning down the little orange pills or sugar cubes and reached instead for the bottle, the mirror or the brown. But the psychedelic tradition was kept alive in the burgeoning 'acid folk' scene, which took us nicely into the free festival scene and the hippie bands resisting the norm.

Lose Your Mind — But Be Sure You're Home For Tea

It's true that, in general, the psychedelic revolution came to the UK late. We didn't have the gradual emergence out of the 1950s Beat Generation to anything like the same extent as they did in the States. Nor did we have the Vietnam War to stir up protest, or such a healthy CIA government-testing program of LSD as they did over there (though there were a few important studies done on British troops which have found themselves onto the internet and become popular on YouTube).[13] In America, there was a larger grassroots development of a jilted generation of poets and writers who slowly adopted the use of the mind-expanding drugs leaking from Leary's set. There were a few notable characters spearheading the way in the UK, but in general the British psychedelic scene emerged instead from a well-established popular culture. Kings Road and Carnaby Street were already exploding with style and popularity by the time LSD came flooding in.

A big part of that flood was the result of Michael Hollingshead, who, in 1965, returned from the States where, since 1961, he had been cavorting with Tim Leary and his large mayonnaise jar of LSD. On his return to London, he brought back with him a huge stack of Leary's guide book, *The Psychedelic Experience*, and set out on a personal mission to 'turn on' the UK. He formed the World Psychedelic Centre in his Belgravia flat in Pont Street, and invited all and sundry (from the trendy set) to learn what the Americans had been doing for the last four years. He had with him 5000 doses of Czechoslovakian LSD, which he dispensed in 300-microgram doses injected into grapes for a host of willing invitees, including Clapton, McCartney, Polanski, Donovan and The Stones.

Psychedelic clubs sprang up all over London, of which the UFO Club in Tottenham Court Road, The Roundhouse in Chalk Farm and the Middle Earth Club in Covent Garden were the most famous.[14] They became the hotspots to watch the jangly groups of the 'British Invasion blues' sound lay down their hard riffs and pick up sitars and beads. All the garb was available from the boutiques of London, including the *uber* fashionable 'Granny Takes a Trip' (immortalized by the Purple Gang's song in 1967), 'Hung on You', 'Biba' and, a little later, 'The Apple Store' (and we are not talking iPads). An influential figure of the day in London was the American producer Joe Boyd whose deft ears brought us Pink Floyd, The Incredible String Band and Fairport Convention. Artistic and literary influences emanated from the Indica Gallery and Bookshop in Soho, owned by John Dunbar, Peter Asher and Barry Miles, and were keenly supported by their neighbour Paul McCartney. It was in the Indica Gallery that John Lennon met Yoko Ono who was displaying her artwork at the time. One of the Ono installations involved climbing a ladder and using a dangling magnifying glass to read a tiny word written on the ceiling. Lennon, who by then already had his eye on Yoko, had told himself that if the message was one of positivity then he and her would hit off. He used the magnifying glass and strained his eyes to see what was written. The word was 'Yes'.

Another centre of cultural influence in the London psychedelic scene was the London Free School in Notting Hill, set up in part by John 'Hoppy' Hopkins in 1965. He and Barry Miles of the Indica Gallery also helped to propagate and disseminate the printed psychedelic word with their paper *International Times*, which, together with *Oz* (founded initially in Sydney by Richard Neville and then had second lysergic outing in London in 1967) brought limited print-run colourful acidic words to the kids in capes tearing round London in their Mini Mokes. For a lovely description of this period of underground publishing history in London check out Richard Neville's recent book *Hippie Hippie Shake*.[15]

Wales, London, Goat-breeding and a WPC Called Julie

In 1977 a major police operation made the UK's biggest ever LSD bust and 'rescued' the streets from six-and-a-half-million doses of the 'killer' drug. This happened after an elaborate undercover police project called Operation Julie, named after one of the female officers working in the team of 28 'undercover hippies', which must have been quite a sight.

The story began nine years earlier when Richard Kemp, a chemist, met American David Solomon who by then was already something of a vintage name on the psychedelic circuit, having written a popular book on drugs earlier in the decade and later founded the British LSD Club. By 1969 Kemp was producing LSD from his flat in West London. By far the hardest thing about making LSD in those days, and still today, is getting hold of the base ingredient, ergotamine tartrate, which, although not itself psychoactive, is also a controlled drug. But Solomon sorted out a sure supply. Another key player in the chain from chemistry set to acid tab included Henry Todd, the distributer. He was joined later by Leaf Fielding, ex-student of Reading University who initially acted as tableter. Also involved was another mysterious character who was strangely both omnipresent and conspicuously absent throughout the whole psychedelic period: Ronald Stark; a man with connections to the world's major producers and suppliers of the drug, The Brotherhood of Eternal Love.

Operations had been moved out of London and into a secluded spot in Wales in 1973. This major LSD production, tableting and distribution network was churning out acid for the UK, European and American markets swimmingly for several years, having stayed completely under the police radar. The acid was being readily swallowed-up at the mushrooming circuit of free festivals that burned all summer long throughout the early seventies in Britain. In 1974, Kemp and Todd fell out. Kemp carried on making acid but didn't have a distribution network. Todd recruited another chemist and their lab in on Seymour Road, London supplied most of the acid taken almost anywhere in the world between 1974–1977: microdots for the UK market and volcanoes (tiny conical-shaped tablets) for the European and wider international scenes. Kemp and his girlfriend, Christine Bott, kept themselves to themselves in their Welsh cottage, playing the part of dropped-out hippies running a small-holding. But, in fact, Kemp was churning out LSD. They grew their own vegetables and generally kept a low profile, though Christine emerged occasionally to parade one of her prize-winning goats at local shows.

In 1975 Richard Kemp was involved in a serious car accident that tragically resulted in the death of a local vicar. When the car was searched the police found a vital clue: a piece of paper that had been ripped up but when put back together spelled the words 'hydrazine hydrate', one of the ingredients necessary for making LSD. The undercover operation was underway.

The police camped out at a nearby Welsh farmhouse and kept watch on Bott and Kemp for almost a year before swooping simultaneously on them and on the Seymour road lab in London. The British LSD ring was busted, and the festival circuit LSD dried up. The cost of a tab went up from 50p to over a pound thereafter.

Most of the main players went to prison for long sentences. Christine Bott had nothing to do with making acid but she was busted for conspiracy. As the other chemist said later: 'I got eleven years for making LSD, Christine got ten nine years for making sandwiches!'

The defence of these LSD producers — and many other suppliers of the drug since — was that theirs was not a major profit-making industry but, rather, a mission to spread the positive effects of their chosen sacrament to the masses, a defence that never works with the judges. Leaf Fielding kindly helped me with this section of the book. Since his release from prison in 1982, he has since gone on to be an educator and philanthropist, setting up a school home for orphaned AIDS children in Malawi. And he has recently released a great book about Operation Julie, *To Live Outside the Law*, which is well worth a read for an insider's view of this fascinating piece of UK memoir.[16]

Haight, Collapse and Blame: It's All LSD's Fault

Of course, as mentioned, by the time London had swallowed the pill in 1967, the Haight-Ashbury area of San Francisco was already in decline. This artsy neighbourhood perched on top of a hill (as is most of San Francisco, depending upon from which angle one is lying) with its wide streets and beautiful wooden houses was where the hippies congregated because it was cheaper than the surrounding San Francisco neighbourhoods. In 1966, when the LSD bomb exploded, tens of thousands of kids, waifs, strays and runaways flooded into the area hoping to find those famous people with flowers in their hair. But by then many of the early pioneers already owned large properties out of town, drifting upwards to the serenity of Marin County or south to LA, where we later saw the move away from psychedelia and the emergence of the singer-songwriter introspection — a natural 'come-down' from the trip.

It seems the hippies were unable to stop the war, which grumbled on with increasing casualties into the mid seventies (when will we learn? — Bush, Reagan, Thatcher, Blair). LSD was made illegal everywhere in 1966 and soon became maligned by 'The Man' as public enemy number one, blamed for the total moral collapse of the idealistic 1950s vision of the American family and the American Dream. The shopping malls had won. Charles Manson's grizzly version of psychedelic reality ended in a horrific bloodbath with the murders at the Polanski residence. The part LSD played in this was obviously seized upon by the media and used as justification why acid was a machination of the devil. Polarisation of the issue allowed politicians to deflect attention from their own killing spree in South East Asia and blame the whole of society's degeneration on a humble molecule derived from mouldy rye.

Timothy Leary was convicted of two very minor cannabis offences and, by 1969, was on the run from the authorities, who were determined to get his guts one way or the other for spoiling the kids' saccharin youth. Nixon dubbed Leary 'The Most Dangerous Man in America' and, in 1970, he was jailed for *30 years* for the possession of two dead roaches. He rightly escaped from jail in an elaborate plot (which absolutely must be made into a film some day) involving The Black Panthers, The Weathermen and those international purveyors of underground acid, The Brotherhood of Eternal Love. Travelling in various disguises and with both formal and informal political and cultural asylum from many sympathetic — and a few unsympathetic — offers of help from Algeria to Beirut, Switzerland to Kabul, and eventually London, found himself then back into the clutches of the authorities in the USA.

The sixties was over, and to quote again from Danny in *Withnail and I:* 'The greatest decade in the history of mankind is coming to an end, man, and as Presuming Ed here has so consistently pointed out, we have failed to paint it black.'

By the early 1970s the Haight neighbourhood had declined into a quagmire of amphetamine and heroin abuse. Homelessness — which today in the Haight (and other districts of the city) has become a national movement worthy of its own sovereign state — quickly set in.

But It's Not All Doom and Gloom

California remained very much the centre of the psychedelic, consciousness-expanding, countercultural cyclone thanks to Esalen, San Francisco and the music scene. But the hippie generation morphed with the times. For those serious-minded folk for whom the psychedelic experience was much more than just a hedonistic thrill, representing, rather, a true journey out of the humdrum consumerism of the growing modernity, they began to organise themselves into new communities with lifestyles centred around communal living.

Just as one-million years ago psychedelics, propagated, maybe, through the galaxy as alien spores clinging onto meteorites from distant stars, brought about human spiritual development by feeding our cave-dwelling ancestors with mind food, catapulting them from cabbage-munchers to sentient god worshippers, so too did the 1960s and the resulting cultural explosion propagate a cultural renaissance of equally important gravity and magnitude. Today's psychedelic community would consider themselves the enlightened 'Children of Aquarius', the Indigo Children. They have drunk the elixir and *know* with absolute certainty that the key to human and, indeed, the entire planet's survival, is through the transcendence of the ordinary limits of human consciousness with the help of psychedelic plants and fungi. There are a great many people who believe this.

LSD, Computer Geeks and Green Activists: A New Age of Social Enlightenment

Today, we have roughly the same genome as we enjoyed 100,000 years ago. And if one subscribes to a purely reductionist viewpoint, this means we have the same physical machinery in our bodies and brains with which to invent our gods, form our religions, develop social structures and work out how to best have relationships with the ones we love and the ones we cannot stand. Despite the external trappings of culture our brains are un-evolved and may as well still be shuffling across the grassy plains of Africa from where we only very recently migrated.

But what *has* evolved is the transmission of ideas and knowledge — information conducted not as genes through DNA, but as memes through collected knowledge recorded in songs, pictures, writing, drama and dance. Psychedelic drugs, and the maelstrom of influence they whipped up in the 1960s and beyond, are the primeval soup in which these memes swim, pushing forward and carrying in their wake information about art, music and fashion.

It is no surprise that the ecology movement sprung directly from the psychedelic scene. A spontaneous and fundamental phenomenon of the psychedelic experience is that of getting close to nature. Under the influence of LSD, one feels in tune with the waves and the wind in the rustle of the trees. These are the feelings that appear to intrinsically entwine one's cells with the cells of those living and natural phenomenon all around. Everything is carried forward in an incessant flow of energy, a vibrational dynamism that feels, at least, as if it is part of something deeper than oneself and not of this age. There is a natural inclination to hark back to archaic times before newspapers, televisions, cars and frappuccinos. In 1953, Huxley lost his mind in the petals of a rose in a vase on the table, gazing dreamily with tear-filled eyes at the pure unadulterated beauty of God, made physical before him. He felt an immediate and natural connection with nature and saw in the flower himself and his place in the world. Yet when Osmond led him out into the Californian sunlight to stroll through the garden he collapsed into hysterical laughter at the sight of the car in the driveway. The absurdity of human invention! How ludicrous and false, how grotesque a mockery of nature is such a thing as a car! It jarred instantly with the feelings of connectivity he had with nature.

So, in the 1960s, the hippies naturally fed into and developed these beliefs. Saving trees, saving whales, vegetarianism, and veganism, hugging trees and recording the screams of flowers as they are picked: these cultural peculiarities, that have since marched with alarming necessity into mainstream political circles as we face the prospect of global ecological disaster, are direct descendants of the LSD experience. Perhaps it is going too far to thank LSD for the Kyoto Agreement (which the US didn't sign up for anyway), but the roots of the green movement certainly owe a lot to the oceanic boundlessness of the psychedelic experience, if you can dig it.

And San Francisco certainly kept its cultural charm, remaining a centre for all things hippie-like — from a commercial point of view at least. In 2010, I went to California for a long weekend to present an update on British Psychedelic Research at the MAPS Conference in San Jose. But I ended up becoming happily stranded, unable to get out even if I had wanted to because of a most generous volcanic explosion from Eyjafjallajökull in Iceland. I stayed in the Red Victorian Hotel on Haight Street — a classic San Franciscan Victorian building, now home to Sami's World Peace Center and representative of all things hippie. I had a wonderful time playing my tunes in the bar for Sami and the staff, and staying in the 'Summer of Love' room for 14 days. By complete coincidence, my April stay also took in the famous annual '4/20' celebration in Golden Gate Park, which saw thousands of modern-day hippies congregate on 'Hippie Hill' dancing to reggae under clouds of smoke, giving me a little taste of what it might have been like back in 1967. Thank you Eyjafjallajökull for that.

It's Not All Over Yet

In the late 1970s and early 1980s, there were still bands emerging from the post-punk era, which harped back to the sounds and the drugs of the 1960s for their inspiration. One of the first bands I ever knew and owned the recordings of was The Soft Boys, courtesy of my sister's then boyfriend, the bass player. They were formed in Cambridge around the enigmatic front-man Robyn Hitchcock, were influenced by 'the four B's' — Beatles, Barrett, Byrds and Beefheart — and their jangly tunes took their listeners back to the 1960s. The genre of 'neo-psychedelia' endured throughout the 1980s with many other bands like Echo and the Bunnymen and Teardrop Explodes emerged on the fringes of 'goth' music and certainly burned a flame for the creative imagination offered by LSD (not that I realised it at the time). But what really brought back all of the culture of the 1960s into the 1980s in all its Technicolor glory was a different molecule altogether, one based not around the tryptamine molecule, but around that of another endogenous brain chemical: phenethylamine.

Ecstasy is Upon Us

In 1988 the UK witnessed a new cultural phenomenon: the rave scene. The drug ecstasy (3,4 — methylenedioxymethamhetamine, or MDMA) became prevalent at large music events, where it's stimulant and mildly hallucinogenic effects were favoured for all-night dancing. The drug has remained immensely popular ever since. Now in the UK around 500,000 people take ecstasy every weekend and over 100 million tablets are consumed annually.[17]

MDMA was first synthesized and patented by the German pharmacological company Merck in 1912. The original intention was that it could be an appetite suppressant for the German army but it never went into the mass production stage. It is interesting to imagine what might have happened in the next two world wars had it actually gone in that direction!

Instead, MDMA was shelved and little more was mentioned about it until the mid fifties, when it resurfaced again alongside a host of other psychotropic drugs being tested by the US military as possible 'truth serums' or weapons of war. At this time, the CIA had a secret operation called MK-ULTRA, in which they tested hundreds of substances, including psychedelic drugs such as LSD on hosts of people in dangerous and unethical circumstances. There are reports of agents giving people drugs without the subjects knowing they had been dosed in order that the agents could watch them surreptitiously. Suffice to say neither LSD nor MDMA made much progress when used in this way by the army. The subjective effects of the psychedelic drugs can become meaningless and unpredictable when no attention is paid to set and setting.

The 1960s drug culture came and went with very little mention of MDMA — the majority of hippies preferring LSD. There was some limited use of the methylated amphetamine MDA, which has similar properties to MDMA, though less empathogenic and longer-lasting. Again, we can only wonder what the cultural, artistic, political and social landscape might have looked like had MDMA been discovered in large quantities in the 1960s instead of LSD; maybe the rave scene of the 1990s would have come early. Woodstock with bleeps?

The Grandfather of MDMA Meets His Grandson for the First Time

In 1967 Alexander 'Sasha' Shulgin was introduced to MDMA by one of his graduate students. Shulgin was an organic chemistry graduate from Harvard who had since worked for the chemical company Dow, where he was very successful. He left Dow in 1965 to pursue his own private business testing drug samples for the DEA. Impressed by MDMA, which he called his 'low-cal Martini' Shulgin continued to take the drug himself — together with whatever new chemical invention he had cooked up that month in his laboratory — with a small group of chosen friends throughout the late 1960s and 1970s. This monthly study group, in which he and his friends methodically tested his new psychedelic discoveries, has become a thing of legend, and Sasha wrote a great book about the experiments, *Tihkal*. Shulgin developed a neat system of rating scales to judge the effectiveness of his new creations, which many aspiring psychonauts still use widely today. Check out any 'trip reports' on *Bluelight* or *Erowid* to see Shulgin's rating scale in action, which rates the drugs' effects from Plus One (+), which is a just noticeable effect, to Plus Four (++++), which is a full-blown spiritual experience.[18]

In 1976 Shulgin developed a new method of synthesis for MDMA, thus bypassing the Merck patent, and then introduced it to psychotherapist Leo Zeff. At this time Zeff was a retired psychedelic psychotherapist who had given up his work with LSD some years earlier, disheartened that he could no longer use it in his practice. But as soon as he experienced MDMA he came out of retirement and began travelling around the States and Europe telling hundreds of people about the drug. Many of these converts went on to use the drug themselves as a tool for psychotherapy. As described in chapter two, it is impossible to ignore the potential that MDMA has for psychotherapy. The unique effects of the drug are almost as if it was invented for this purpose. A new legal alternative to LSD for psychedelic therapy had been discovered.

MDMA Becomes Too Popular, Gets Banned and MAPS is Born

What happened next is broadly similar to the path taken by LSD, in that what had been developed through careful and judicious study in the clinic could not help leaking into the wider community. By 1980 there were reports of this new substance turning up in trendy Dallas nightclubs, which, at this time (as the TV show *Dallas* will bear testament to), was a burgeoning culture of wealth and decadence. Some described the acceptance of this new drug (then called 'Adam') to be 'more popular than cocaine'. Being primarily a stimulant, like cocaine, but with a delightful added mild psychedelic effect, it was perfect for partying and dancing. People began calling it 'empathy', in line with the positive mood effects when used clinically.[19]

Of course, as soon as it became apparent that mass interest was around the corner the next step was inevitable. In 1984 the DEA took steps to ban the then still legal MDMA. It called for emergency legislation to have the drug placed in Schedule One, which meant it was defined as having 'no medical uses'. The small but vociferous band of psychotherapists who by then had developed their effective and growing psychotherapy regimes with MDMA protested against this measure. A hearing took place and the judge took testimony from both sides. Against MDMA the scientists hired by the government submitted claims about it's danger, suggesting it had a high toxicity profile (such claims have since been discredited); and in favour of MDMA the therapists argued their case that it can be used safely and can relive many forms of mental disorder. The judge saw reason and placed the drug in Schedule Three (equivalent to Class C in the UK), which meant it was available to bona fide therapists to use with caution. But the government/DEA overruled the judge (which, let's face it, makes a mockery of the judicial process if governments can do such a thing) and MDMA was placed firmly into Schedule One, where it has stayed since.

For those therapists who had held such promise for this new drug as a tool for psychotherapy there was much disappointment. A pressure group was set up to strive for more research to try to convince the regulatory authorities that there were important medical uses for the drug. From this group emerged Rick Doblin and the formation of the Multidisciplinary Association for Psychedelic Studies (MAPS). MAPS has since campaigned furiously for evidence-based research to fight the corner for clinical MDMA and other psychedelic drugs. But it has been an uphill battle all the way, caught as it is in the Catch-22 situation whereby there is not enough data out there to support MDMA as a medicine so it remains banned, and because it is banned it is very difficult to get a license to carry out the studies to prove it is safe in order to lift the ban. It was this frustration that has dogged MDMA research for the last 30 years, though is now thankfully beginning to shift.

Banning MDMA Gives Birth to Ecstasy and Rave

Meanwhile, in the early eighties MDMA was picking up as a recreational drug. Legend has it that around this time an entrepreneurial dealer of MDMA decided that the name 'Empathy' would not be such a good selling point, so changed it to Ecstasy, which clearly did the trick.

In the mid eighties it came to Europe via a small band of followers of the Indian style-guru, Bhagwan 'Osho' Shree Rajneesh.[20] Osho's American commune in Oregon had been shut down in 1984 and his followers had disseminated across the globe, many going to Ibiza, which by now was a popular hippie hang out for those still coming down from the 1960s. The Osho-ites spread their message of love and sex through the use of meditation and MDMA and, by 1987, when DJs Danny Rampling, Paul Oakenfold and Nicky Holloway went there for a holiday and experienced the embryonic nightlife, the links between ecstasy and house music had well and truly been made.[21]

The DJs returned to the UK and set up the club *Shoom* in South London, which gave birth to rave music and took the movement nicely into the so-called Second Summer of Love, occurring in 1988. A double-stranded approach to the use of

MDMA meant the craze sped off in two rather separate directions: one being the dance scene and the other being the sounds coming out of Manchester propagated by the likes of The Stone Roses and The Happy Mondays — whose drug of choice was the same little pills with stamped pictures of doves that were being sold to the ravers in Ibiza and London. Ecstasy became incredibly popular in the UK in the last years of the eighties and by the early nineties was second only to cannabis as the young people's illegal drug of choice.

Raves sprang up everywhere. Initially they were small-scale collective party gatherings born out of the 1960s Free Festival circuit. The Free Festivals had rolled along throughout the 1960s, fuelled by a enormous production of LSD in the mid seventies and the continuing rock scene. Massive gatherings at Stonehenge took place every year and attracted a more and more diverse crowd as punk influenced the crowds. The Peace Convoy provided an opportunity for free-spirited folk to take to the road and live a itinerant lifestyle, travelling from party to party and rejecting the grimness of the 1970s British existence.

Modern Raving, Festivals and Shamanism: Come Together

Many scholars, sixties hippies and contemporary ravers alike have compared the modern concept of partying on psychedelic drugs to the archaic work of the shaman. Both occur mainly at night, when the shadows and hidden crevices of the dark jungle night is mimicked by the darkened corridors of a nightclub or festival scene; both encourage the imagination to fill in the gaps and expand the possibilities of what might be out there looking on; and both raving and shamanistic rituals tend to go on all night long: participants are definitely in it for the long haul. It is not like having a couple of stiff of drinks; there is a far greater commitment than that.

Shamans and DJs both rely on the trance-inducing qualities of repetitive music. Beats from drums that loop over and over again, drawing the listener in, removing the opportunities for complex melody and inducing a vacant stare into the hidden gaps between the notes. But that is not to say the music is mindless or lacking in beauty; on the contrary, it is these primeval sounds that connect one with nature. Everything is repetitive and cyclical; tribal drumming emphasises this point.

Psychedelic parties have a powerful cohesive, group effect on those experiencing the shared altered state of consciousness, just as they do for the village participants in a shamanic ceremony. Participants are not merely being told about *someone else's* experience of the spiritual realms as happens in a traditional church service. Instead, every single person in the room, under the trees or on the dance floor is an active participant up there, in front of Mother Nature, staring Her in the face and directly experiencing the power and wisdom of Her words.

At a rave the shaman is the DJ and MC. He or she is directing the ceremony, leading the crowd along with their breakdowns, the tweaking of the cerebral EQs and controlling the lights. Strobes flash and the smoke machine pumps out another gush of mind-clouding material onto the dance floor as directed by the Master of Ceremonies. Everyone is safely in his or her hands. The DJ will challenge you. They will not let you get away lightly; you are there to experience the peaks of the drug's effects and this will not be a walk in the park — if it were there would be nothing to learn from the experience. But you know they will keep you safe and keep your eyes open so you will not miss a beat.

The group psychedelic experience at a rave or in a festival is the modern day Western version of a shamanistic community ritual. It is more than just a hedonistic act, more than a mere 'acute confusional state'. It requires hard work, diligence and careful guidance. And when these factors are followed it may result in spiritual and personal growth, and play an important role in social cohesion and stability.

Kids on E

For an excellent firsthand description of a young person taking his or her pioneer ecstasy tablet and experiencing the positivity, the highs and the lows of their first rave, try a careful listening to the song Weak Become Heroes by the band *The Streets*. Few artists describe the impact of the rave scene on UK youth better.

In the UK, it all came together big time at an infamous gathering of tribes for the Castlemorton Common Festival on May Bank Holiday in 1992. It was here we saw a coming together of Ibiza ravers with the hardened crusty travellers from the old Stonehenge-Peace Convoy-Free Festival circuit of the 1980s; these disparate tribes combined for a five day anti-authority event, united by ecstasy and dance music. The skanky psychedelic garb of the travellers met the trendy London neoprene of the ravers head-on and everyone realised they had a common purpose: to stay up all weekend long, peak and dance. While the post-punk travellers' favourite intoxicant of the past had been psilocybin mushrooms, amphetamine and high-strength canned beer both groups shared their love of cannabis and MDMA, and the marriage made in Castlemorton was born. The huge illegal party raged for five days and nights whilst a bemused local population looked on incredulously. The police were unable to stop the event for five days and it eventually made front pages everywhere and was probably the single most important event that lead to the eventual Criminal Justice Bill in the UK.[22]

DJ sound systems took over everywhere in the nineties, such was the general dross on offer in the popular music scene. Dance music rarely crept into the mainstream except in its most insipid form. The parties were in the custody of the kids and always one step ahead of the police.

Demonization of Ecstasy

Over the course of the 1990s, ecstasy became the new public enemy number one (it seems like there always has to be one — not sure what it is now. . . bankers perhaps, which, I suppose, is a progression in a the right direction!). But things started going wrong, just as they had with LSD twenty years earlier. The quality of ecstasy tablets plummeted and people began using nastier drugs. There were several high-profile tragic deaths of young people who took E for the first time in unsafe circumstances, and far too many people were over-indulging.

What happened next, quite inevitably, was that rave went mainstream, perhaps best characterized by the London group The Shaman, who sampled Terence McKenna's drones above a trancy beat. The band stormed the charts with 'Ebenezer Goode' in 1993 ('E's are good, E's are good. . . . He's Ebenezer Goode!'.[23]

Much to the chagrin of the UK drinks industry, kids in clubs stopped drinking booze and chose to supplement their E's with bottles of water instead. The drinks industry fought back with it's development of 'Alco pops' — an obvious tip in the direction of the 'instant hit' but applied to ethanol rather than MDMA. This was a successful drive and we have seen the UK drinking culture climb back to its ferocious position again since then. The state-sanctioned legitimate alcohol peddlers have always been keen to put down illegal drugs. That is the trouble with keeping drugs illegal: there is no money to be made from it for governments.

Then, in 1994, the British government made its greatest hit back at rave with the introduction of the Criminal Justice Bill, with its famous quote describing electronic music as 'sounds wholly or predominantly characterised by the emission of a succession of repetitive beats'. The new legislation meant police had increased powers of 'stop and search', and could more easily break up gatherings of people and confiscate sound systems without having to gain advance consent. My colleagues/friends and I marched through London in our best rave regalia and partied all day up against police barricades in Hyde Park in October that year. It was a true 'fight for your right to party' moment, dancing to mobile sound systems in scenes reminiscent of the sixties, but to no avail. The Man had won, again.

MDMA Research On the Ropes and Labels
On the Wrong Bottles

As the 1990s drew on, Rick Doblin and the Multidisciplinary Association for Psychedelic Studies, MAPS, was struggling like mad to re-establish psychedelics' role in medicine. The demonization of ecstasy was effectively grounding all research just as the backlash against LSD in the mid sixties did for psychedelic research 30 years earlier. And in much the same way as for LSD, the illegalisation of ecstasy did nothing to reduce its recreational use but was perfect at stopping bona fide medical research.

Reagan's presidency between 1981 and 1989 carried on Nixon's all out War On Drugs just as blindly, steamrolling its way through the media and the courts, blocking Doblin at every opportunity. Reagan was followed by George H. W. Bush, 1989–1993, and he was certainly no better.

Between 1986 and 1988 Doblin submitted to the FDA (the Food and Drinks Authority, the American version of the ethics committee required to conduct medical drug research) five different applications for permission to conduct human research with MDMA and all five were rejected.[24] The FDA said there was too much risk of neurotoxicity from MDMA. But Doblin persisted. He knew the rejections were not for objective scientific reasons but because of an underlying cultural prejudice. The authorities simply could not see, or did not *want* to see, that an illegal recreational drug could have any clinical benefit. It would send the wrong message to the kids. Doblin was rightly concerned that the same thing that happened with LSD at the end of the sixties was happening again with MDMA. A socio-politically motivated cultural backlash was threatening to stop medical research in its tracks and the result was that patients lost out. This could not be allowed to happen again. Surely the only message to send is the truth? But MAPS was caught in the imposed Catch 22. There was an insufficient amount of data, and MAPS wasn't allowed to go out and get it.

In the late eighties and early nineties, MAPS continued to do what it could, funding animal toxicity and Phase One human studies at Stanford and Johns Hopkins Universities in the States. Then Doblin's perseverance began to pay off. In 1992 Dr. Charles Grob, Professor of Child and Adolescent Psychiatry at UCLA, submitted a protocol for a clinical MDMA study on patients with end-stage cancer. The FDA started to see sense, and said they would consider this protocol only after a further Phase-One safety study was conducted on MDMA to test it's toxicity at the doses proposed for therapy. The safety study was approved and subsequently completed in 1995. It demonstrated — just as everyone at MAPS expected — that MDMA did not present any significant risks to humans at the doses and patterns of doses proposed for psychotherapy. The FDA, however, remained cautious for the rest of the decade and continued with their bureaucracy that made it very difficult for Grob's study to progress.

Meanwhile in Spain, Dr. Jose Carlos Bouso, who has also been planning a MAPS-sponsored MDMA for PTSD study, eventually got approval for this in 1999, and it got underway in 2000. But just over a year after starting Bouso's Spanish study it began to falter. After just six of the planned 29 patients on the study have had their initial dosing with MDMA the Spanish government — fuelled by a political backlash influenced by negative media pressure — bears heavily on Bouso and the study is shut down. It is 2002, some 17 years since MDMA was banned, and clinical research is still a very distant dream. Everything seems to be against the clinical study of MDMA. There is just too much erroneous negative pressure filling the newspapers, augmented by media scare stories about reckless ravers and international drug cartels. Despite the fact these issues have nothing to do with the medical use of MDMA therapy, governments everywhere dare not back the research for fear of unwanted political fallout. And this attitude of fear and bias is even infiltrating into the scientific community, with a host of methodologically unsound and even, possibly, downright scandalously flawed data supporting the entrenched position of the governments who wish to continue their War On Drugs — even when it flies in the face of medical necessity.

As mentioned earlier, there was that famous incident in 2002, which illustrates well the farcical debate, when Dr. George Ricaurte, working for a US-government-sponsored MDMA project, published a study that apparently unequivocally demonstrated severe neurotoxicity in primates who had been given only moderate amounts of MDMA. The study appeared in the highly influential journal *Science* and Ricaurte's damning results were beamed all over the world. Here was the smoking gun. The international media and governments jumped on the story and used it as clear justification for their heavy restrictions on MDMA research and on those troublesome clubbers. But then, in 2003, it transpired that Ricaurte's research had been highly inaccurate. His team had not given their primates MDMA at all, but rather *methamphetamine* — a highly toxic compound that bore no resemblance to MDMA. Although Ricaurte subsequently retracted his study from *Science* and offered an apology, the damage was done and governments clung on to that smoking gun for many years — perhaps they still do. I am no conspiracy theorist but Doblin has certainly continued to pursue exactly what went on there. It is not known whether either someone in Ricaurte's lab switched the bottles by accident or on purpose, or whether the DEA themselves were involved at the original source of the drug. One way or another the erroneous result caused an enormous amount of damage to genuine MDMA research and the apparent 'accident' fitted in well to the malevolent political agenda against MDMA.[25]

Doblin Meets Mithoefer at a Conference for the Spiritual Vine

In 2000 Doblin met Michael Mithoefer at an ayahuasca conference in San Francisco sponsored by Leary's old colleague Ralph Metzner. Mithoefer, a psychiatrist from South Carolina with a lifelong interest in MDMA and an experienced practitioner with cases of severe PTSD, believed strongly that MDMA might offer a desperately needed new therapeutic approach for his patients. Unfortunately, by this point Dr. Grob's study looking at patients with end-stage cancer was not happening at all, due to the DEA's continued barriers to using MDMA so he decided to use psilocybin instead. He went on to produce a ground-breaking clinical study with psilocybin, which we will come to later.

By the turn of the new millennium, dance music, and ecstasy use, had moved to a new level. Perhaps because of the Criminal Justice Act, what used to happen in small clubs and dingy warehouses at an underground level is now filling arenas and supporting a whole legitimate industry on both sides of the Atlantic. In 2000, the ubiquitous direct drive Technics 1210 turntable, the standard hardware set-up for any self-respecting disc jockey, was outselling guitars for the first time as the teenage Christmas present of choice. Vinyl was back on the shelves and now everyone it seems wants to be a DJ. MDMA had saved the vinyl record industry.

Things Start Looking Up for MDMA Research

With the turn of the new millennium, Mithoefer and Doblin gained approval for the PTSD study and over many further years of red tape and headaches it got underway. However, recruitment and enrolment remain slow in the face of so many bureaucratic restrictions. The researchers apply to the review board to make an amendment, wishing to add a third MDMA session to the course of therapy, which takes a full 3 years to get approval but they keep going, slowly seeing 37 patients through the treatment protocol.

In 2005, I wrote my first editorial for the *British Journal of Psychiatry* on the state of international psychedelic research.[26] Although the movement was in full swing in the States by this stage, I felt disheartened that, for the vast majority of my generation of British psychiatrists, it was still an unknown subject. Rick Doblin was supportive of my work and encouraged me to cast the net wider to try to bring on board more psychiatrists from the UK. Through my *British Journal of Psychiatry* paper, and while still in Oxford, I met Amanda Feilding. In 2007, after my work came to the attention of David Nutt, I put Nutt and Mithoefer together, and, in his role as president of the European College of Neuropsyhcopharmacology (ECNP), Nutt invited us both to talk on the state of psychedelic research at the annual meeting in Vienna and we met again when I invited him over to the UK, together with Charlie Grob, to speak at a symposium in Liverpool I was chairing at the Royal College of Psychiatrists Annual Conference in 2009. That symposium was approved for the College by one of the UK's leading psychiatrists specialising in PTSD, Dr. Jonathan Bisson from Cardiff University, and this moment would prove to be another important stepping stone in the story of MDMA research in the UK — but none of us knew it just yet.

Then, in 2010, Michael Mithoefer's study was fully written up. I was invited to review the paper for the *Journal of Psychopharmacology*, for which David Nutt was the chief editor. The data was in. MDMA Therapy could be delivered safely and effectively to treat PTSD. The paper was approved and the world's first human clinical MDMA study was published — a whole 35 years after it was inappropriately banned in the first place. Rick Doblin, whose dream to see this happen dates back to 1985, deserves a Nobel Prize for his perseverance. His work has only just begun.

CHAPTER 6

Psychedelic Creativity

Measuring the Influence of Psychedelics on Creativity

It is perhaps no surprise that John Lennon, after taking LSD, thought George Harrison's heavily chimney-stacked Berkshire mansion resembled a giant submarine. LSD does stuff like that. The link between psychedelics and creativity is ancient, and, as Terence McKenna would have us believe, these peculiar compounds could account not only for brief excursions into creativity during the course of the acute intoxication with the drug, but also for the entire development of human consciousness itself. Indeed, looking at the role LSD played in so many facets of human life in the sixties, one might conclude that never before have so many fields of human endeavour, from art and architecture, to fashion, music and design, owed so much to such a small molecule.

Certainly, human creativity is difficult to define and measure. And it is such an important cognitive process that it becomes an interesting challenge for modern scientific exploration. There are clear similarities between the typical traits of creative people and the subjective psychological characteristics of the psychedelic drug experience.[1] This phenomenon — which may seem obvious to some people but ludicrous to others — was studied in a number of small trials and case studies in the 1960s but results were inconclusive, and the quality of these studies by modern research standards was merely anecdotal.

Nevertheless, with today's current renaissance in psychedelic drug research, now is the time to revisit these studies with contemporary research methods and neuroimaging. Like many aspects of modern psychedelic research, this is a study just waiting to happen. But the majority of today's contemporary psychedelic studies, as in the 1960s, focus mainly on the drugs' potential clinical applications. Modern research that re-opens avenues for experiments with less obvious clinical applications may in turn add to our understanding of the aesthetic and creative elements of the human brain.

Creativity, Psychedelics and the Human Brain

The well-documented but erroneous 'left-brain versus right-brain' model of brain functioning polarises and oversimplifies an individual's cognitive and creative skills as either artistic, at the expense of language and mathematics, or vice versa. But modern functional neuroimaging challenges this popularly held belief and instead provides a three-factor anatomical model of creativity that focuses on interactions between the temporal lobes, frontal lobes and limbic system. The neuroscientist Robin Carhart-Harris at Imperial University has shown the direct role psilocybin has in activating the area of the brain associated with the retrieval of emotional memories, providing an immediate link between creativity and expanded levels of consciousness. This finding fits with the known observation that creative thinking requires more than just a general intelligence and specific knowledge, but also the ability to develop alternative solutions to a single question, requiring divergent thinking and the ability to form novel ideas.[2]

Many psychedelic explorers come to entertain the view that mind/consciousness is present throughout the universe, and it is not just the by-product of brain activity. A reductionist point of view, on the other hand, postulates that highly creative individuals are able to store extensive specialised knowledge in their temporoparietal cortex, be capable of divergent thinking mediated by the frontal lobe and, crucially, be able to modulate the activity of the locus coeruleus (which fires in response to novel stimuli — and also under the influence of the drug LSD) via the norepinephrine system 'to understand and express novel orderly relationships'.[2]

Since the Renaissance creativity has often been measured in terms of examining the output of so-called creators. The sheer volume of works by Da Vinci and Michelangelo are frequently quoted as testament to their creative geniuses. However, defining objective measures for the process of creativity is notoriously difficult, especially when taking into account the subjective nature of an individual's aesthetic appreciation of a particular creation. It is arguable, of course, that by definition creativity defies measurement, because all tests have predetermined correct answers and originality is a requirement of creativity — implying that any 'correct' answer in a creativity test could not be creative.[3]

The psychological experience induced in humans under the influence of psychedelic drugs is multifarious and idiosyncratic. Nevertheless, a broad range of common characteristics are frequently identified. Alongside the alterations in the user's perceptions, changes in the emotions and expansion of thought and identity a particular feature of the experience has special relevance to the creative process. The psychedelic experience is one of a general increase in complexity and openness, such that the usual ego-bound restraints that allow humans to accept given, preconceived ideas about themselves and the world around them are necessarily challenged. Another important feature is the tendency for users to assign unique and novel meanings to their experience, together with an appreciation that they are part of a bigger, cosmic oneness. These experiences — like those features of spirituality, which were described earlier in the book — are fundamental and arise spontaneously for any users of psychedelic drugs, regardless of any pre-experience or social influence. The evidence for the universal nature of such experiences comes from the multi-cultural similarities of the experiences of users of psychedelic drugs throughout the world.

Unsurprisingly, there are many anecdotal examples of artists and writers describing the use of psychedelic drugs, such as LSD, to enhance the creative process (and a similar number of such accounts disputing this suggestion). The use of drugs to enhance artistic creativity is not new, illustrated when the Roman poet Ovid said, 'There is no poetry among water drinkers'. There are examples of pre-historic art from all around the world that use optical illusions or entoptic phenomena to enhance the visual experience. This observation has been recently studied by a group of researchers including the anthropologist Luis E. Luna from the Research Centre for the Study of Psychointegrator Plants, Visionary Arts, and Consciousness, located in Brazil. Their paper, 'Enhancement of creative expression and entoptic phenomena as an after-effect of repeated ayahuasca administration', which I reviewed and approved for the *Journal of Psychopharmacology*, is awaiting publication.[4] In it, they examine the frequency of entopic shapes reported as emerging in the visual fields of users of ayahuasca. More studies of this sort will undoubtedly appear in coming years as we delve ever deeper into the quagmire of thought that links neuroscience with art. David Luke at the University of Greenwich, a passionate and informed proponent of psychedelics, creativity and psi phenomena, is a keen supporter of this direction of study.[5]

Art, Music and Psychedelic Creativity

The links between artwork and the prehistoric use of psychedelic drugs is well established; it is described in the artwork of many ancient cultures from Ireland, Africa France, and South America to as far afield as Siberia and the Arctic Circle. The use of opium (while not usually credited as a psychedelic drug) to influence creativity is also well recognised. Thomas De Quincey described the pleasures and the pitfalls of taking opium in early-nineteenth-century England, and the romantic poet Samuel Taylor Coleridge reported the vivid imagery of the opium experience in his poem *Kubla Khan*, as did Alexandre Dumas Pere and Alfred Lord Tennyson.[6] In the twentieth century, the French poet and playwright Antonin Artaud used opium extensively, as well as the peyote cactus.[7] More recent examples of artists using psychedelic drugs include Henri Michaux, the Belgian-born French painter, journalist and poet, who at the age of 56 started using mescaline and cannabis, and wrote about his experiences in his later works.[8] And, as we have seen, Huxley's famous account of his mescaline experience in 1953 secured his place as a centrally revered figure for the subsequent cultural drug revolution that followed.

Since the 1960s, the volume of modern Western art and music that attributes its influences to the psychedelic drugs is vast. Some such artists and musicians openly proclaim themselves to be 'psychedelic artists', whereas many others will frequently acknowledge the influence that psychedelic drug experiences have had on their work. One such piece of psychedelic drug-influenced artwork even recently appeared on the front cover of the *British Journal of Psychiatry* in homage to the discoverer of LSD, Dr. Albert Hofmann. It was a work by the visionary psychedelic photographer Dean Chamberline, which I submitted in 2006 to celebrate Albert Hofmann's 100th birthday.[9]

Some of the finest and most original pieces of popular music to come out of the Western world in the last six decades have been directly influenced by the psychedelic experience; indeed, we have already touched upon the vast body of work attributed to LSD that forms the basis of the genre of psychedelic music. Suffice to say, there are hundreds of bands and thousands of tunes — from the briefest punkadelic explosions of cerebral damage to triple-gatefold albums of Prog Rock dirge about pixies, crystals and timeless voids — all of them striving to capture the essence of the psychedelic experience onto crackling vinyl. 'Pure tone poem imagery' is how George Martin described The Beatles' psychedelic period of musical influence.

Studying How Psychedelics Influence Creativity

An attempt to explore the value of the agent LSD in influencing artistic creativity was made in a remarkable long-term series of anecdotal case studies by the American psychiatrist Oscar Janiger.[10] Between 1954 and 1962, he facilitated LSD sessions for almost 1000 people between ages 18 and 81 in a variety of professions, from doctors and nurses, lawyers, housewives and police officers to judges, truckers, students, and the unemployed and retired, including the film star Cary Grant. In contrast to the often highly controlled design of most other psychedelic research of this period, Janiger's experiments were largely unguided and took place in a naturalistic setting — his own home — with a view to exploring what the nature of the 'intrinsic, characteristic LSD response' (if indeed there was one) might be. Unsurprisingly, the volunteer's reports varied widely. Adverse reactions were extremely rare, and the vast majority described the experience as valuable and sustaining. During the course of this work with LSD, two experiential characteristics emerged repeatedly: those of spontaneous spiritual experiences and those where there was a boosting of the subjects' experiences of creativity. These latter observations led Janiger to conduct a parallel study examining the effects of the drug on creativity in a controlled setting.

He subsequently gave LSD to a mixed group of 60 visual artists over a seven-year period, and they produced over 250 drawings that were later analysed by a professor of art history, who compared the artists' work before and after the LSD sessions. Because of the heterogeneity of the population and the aesthetic nature of analysing the results, making objective statements about how LSD effected the artists' creativity is impossible. That said, the drug did appear to enhance certain aspects of the artists' work; namely, there was a tendency towards more expressionistic work, a sharpening of colour, a greater freedom from prescribed mental sets, an increased syntactical organisation, a deeper accessibility of past impressions and a heightened sense of emotional excitement. However, perhaps the most valuable aspect of Janiger's study is the many qualitative reports from the artists themselves, who without exception found the LSD experience artistically and personally profound.

Further experiments in creativity and psychedelics include those of Stanley Krippner in the early 1970s, and a much earlier study by Berlin in 1955 in which four prominent graphic artists were given mescaline and LSD and encouraged to complete paintings under the influence of the drug.[11] A panel of art critics judged their subsequent paintings to have 'greater aesthetic value' than the artist's usual work. In the mid sixties, the American psychologist Frank Barron gave psilocybin to creative individuals and recorded their subjective impressions,[12] and the psychiatrist McGlothlin gave LSD to graduate students who subsequently described a greater appreciation of music and the arts, but no actual increase in creative ability.[13] Many of the creativity psychedelic studies of the 1960s paid little attention to the importance of set and setting, two very important factors, as we have seen, that have been shown to radically alter the outcome of individual's experiences under psychedelic drugs.

A Really Nice Study by James Fadiman and Colleagues

A study in 1966 by Harman and Jim Fadiman from the Institute of Psychedelic Research of San Francisco State College deserves closer attention.[14] The researchers took particular care to select individuals already engaged in creative industries (engineers, theoretical mathematicians, physicists, architects and designers) and 'primed' them with a pre-drug session in which they were encouraged to select problems of a professional interest that required a creative solution. The researchers, who told the subjects that the drug would enhance their creativity and help them to work more productively without distractions, therefore encouraged a very positive mind-set. At the psychedelic sessions (using mescaline) a few days later, subjects were encouraged to work in groups and as individuals to tackle their chosen problems and were subjected to psychometric tests. Afterwards, subjects submitted a written subjective account of their experience and were then interviewed by the researchers eight weeks later. All participants showed enhanced abilities on all tests when under the drug compared with the previous non-drug tests and, in the subjective written accounts, all the participants described subjective enhanced effects of the drug on their creative process. From these qualitative reports the researchers formulated a mechanism by which psychedelic drugs can enhance creativity:

1. Reduced inhibition and reduced anxiety.
2. Improved capacity to restructure problems in a wider context.
3. Increased fluency and flexibility of ideas.
4. Increased visual imagery and fantasy.
5. Increased ability to concentrate.
6. Increased empathy with objects and processes.
7. Increased empathy with people.
8. Subconscious data more accessible.
9. Improved association of dissimilar ideas.
10. Heightened motivation to obtain closure.
11. Improved ability to visualize the completed solution.

Although this study is limited by not being double-blind and placebo-controlled, it reports the power and importance of set and setting, and its potential implications for the creative industries is highly significant.

Commercial and Design Applications for Psychedelic Creativity: LSD Architecture

A better understanding of creativity and how best to enhance it has vast implications for commercial industry. Above and beyond the artistic and neuroscientific interest in the creative process, practically all aspects of modern industry rely to some extent on the concept of product design — particularly in the advertising industry, where creativity is arguably the most important element of success. Despite the enormous amount of money and energy invested in such commercial industries, the scientific concept of how creativity is enhanced is poorly understood. This makes the neuroscientific understanding of these processes particularly relevant.

There have been some notable historical examples of designers using psychedelic drugs to improve their skills. One such example from 1965 is when the architect Kyoshi Izumi was asked to design a psychiatric hospital in Canada and decided to take LSD and perform extensive visits to old mental institutions in an attempt to see the wards in a new light.[15] He found himself terrified by the standard hospital paraphernalia such as the tiles on the walls, the recessed closets and the raised hospital beds. There was no privacy, and the sense of time was nil, because of the absence of clocks and calendars. After his LSD insights, Izumi was able to design what has since been called 'the ideal mental hospital'. The first was built in Yorkton, Saskatchewan, and five others have since been modelled upon it elsewhere in Canada.

From Double-helix DNA to San Franciscan Hippies and Geeks with Mice

Another example of the creative influence of psychedelic drugs — though possibly more psychedelic legend than reality — comes from the alleged use of low doses of LSD by the Nobel Prize winner Francis Crick, who discovered the double-helix structure of the DNA molecule in Cambridge in the 1950s. The drug was freely available at that time as a tool for psychotherapy and Crick, who was a well-known admirer of Aldous Huxley and went on to campaign for the legalisation of cannabis in the 1960s, could have easily accessed the drug.

A well-established incidence of psychedelic drug-induced creativity from the scientific community comes from the Nobel-Prize-winning chemist Dr. Kary Mullis, the inventor of the Polymerase Chain Reaction process, who is quoted as saying: 'Would I have invented PCR if I hadn't taken LSD? I seriously doubt it. . . . I could sit on a DNA molecule and watch the polymers go by. I learnt that partly on psychedelic drugs'. A further striking example of psychedelic drug-enhanced creativity in industry comes from the computer industry in California. The liberal atmosphere and loose approach to creativity fostered by the 1960s use of LSD on the West Coast of the United States spawned a population a creative post-hippie entrepreneurs. Pioneers such as Steve Jobs and Steve Wozniak, founders of the

Apple computer industry, were both products of the LSD-fuelled counterculture setting out to turn computers into a means for freeing minds and information.[16]

Clinical Applications for Psychedelic Creativity: Autism

Clinically, how can we use this creativity phenomenon associated with psychedelics? Perhaps the most obvious area is that of autism. Patients with autism are often unable to see the intrinsic and abstract connectivity between people and objects. And one of the central features of the psychedelic experience is the improved ability to find new meaning in and see associations between objects through feeling as if one were participating in an enhanced part of the abstract connectivity of the universe. Although these are subjective effects enhanced only acutely during the psychedelic experience, they are experiences enjoyed by most people to a lesser degree at all times, but in autism, such experiences are frequently impaired.

This phenomenon was explored in the early part of the 1960s in a small number of studies using LSD on children with autism, as previously discussed in chapter five of this book. One study looked at subjects between 6 and 10 years old, all severe cases of autism who had failed to respond to other forms of treatment. Consistent effects of the psychedelic drugs included improved speech in otherwise muted patients, a greater emotional responsiveness to other children and adults, increased positive mood with frequent smiling and laughter, and decreases in obsessive-compulsive behaviour. After a long hiatus, there are now researchers looking again at the role for psychedelics as a treatment for autism. The researcher Alicia Danforth and others working with MAPS have begun looking at designing such a study. In particular, the drug MDMA, a known empathogenic drug, is being researched as a tool to enhance psychotherapy for people with Autism Spectrum Disorder.

But all research into the links between psychedelics and creativity struggle with measuring the extent to which creativity is being altered. It is often difficult to get meaningful data because subjects frequently become engrossed in the subjective aspects of the drug experience and lose interest in the tasks presented by the investigators. Understandably, psychological tests are often seen as absurd or irrelevant by the subjects, illustrated well by this quote from the psychologist Arthur Kleps:

> If I were to give you an IQ test and during the administration one of the walls of the room opened up, giving you a vision of the blazing glories of the central galactic suns, and at the same time your childhood began to unreel before your inner eye like a three-dimension colour movie, you too would not do well on an intelligence test.[17]

The Future Looks Creative for Psychedelic Research

With psychedelic research's current renaissance, the current political climate is beneficial for exploring the therapeutic possibilities of such drugs that have hitherto been considered off limits simply because they have been used recreation-ally. In recent years, we have seen Walter Pahnke's famous Marsh Chapel Experi-ment re-created by Roland Griffiths at Johns Hopkins University, provide objective evidence of the spiritual experience under the influence of psychedelic drugs. Another interesting area for the revisiting of research would be for some brave researcher to recreate the previously mentioned study by Harman and Fadiman to provide similar data on the objective association between creativity and psy-chedelics to the neuroscientific community. As mentioned, such a study could also have some great implications for clinical and commercial sectors of society. In the meantime, however, we'll just have to take John's word for it that George's house looked like a submarine.

CHAPTER 7

Modern Uses of Natural Plant and Fungi Psychedelics

If we are to progress, we have to break away from our restrictive Western view of what functions and what doesn't when it comes to improving our individual and societal health. The apparently instinctive model of unbridled greed simply does not work and it *will* kill us unless we experience a global transcendence of our current level of consciousness — not necessarily spiritually but, certainly, socially and behaviourally. This need to go beyond current attitudes to health, politics and the organisation of society is no longer a fringe point of view held by the bearded and beaded, but, in recent years, has rather become the talk of mainstream politics.[1] Our relentless destruction of the non-Western world over the last two thousand years, and particularly through industrialization in the last 150, is shooting us in our Nike Air clad feet, when what we really need to do is re-learn how to slip off our sandals and start feeling the sand between our toes again.

We know for certain that the sacramental use of magic mushrooms has been going strong in the last 5000 years of recorded human history and there is no reason to believe it hasn't played an equally central role in human life since the dawn of humans themselves. Indeed, if the graph is extrapolated backwards from 5000 years ago, there is plenty of evidence to suggest sacrificial mushroom consumption was more, rather than less, widespread the further back one goes.

Wasson All the Fuss About?

Perhaps an even more influential event than Huxley's 1953 excursion into his 'archipelagos of the mind' on mescaline is Gordon Wasson's 1957 excursion to Mexico in search of the psilocybin mushroom. This truly deserves the credit for kick-starting the massive cultural changes of the 1960s.

The American Robert Gordon Wasson was, believe it or not, yet another character from psychedelic history with a wide range of esoteric interests. And, like many others in the field, once the subject of psychedelic drugs seduced him they changed the direction of his life thereafter. He was initially a banker, the vice president of J. P. Morgan & Co. no less, who developed a sideline interest in mushrooms through his Russian wife, who was, incidentally, a child psychiatrist.

In 1955 the pair travelled to Mexico to carry out field research on the cultural use of fungi and discovered the locals using magic mushrooms as part of their spiritual practice. Wasson became the first Western outsider to participate in a psilocybin mushroom ceremony when given the sacrament by the *Mazatec curandera* (local shaman) Maria Sabina.[2] When Wasson returned to the USA and published his results for *Life* magazine in 1957, along with pictures taken by the photographer Allan Richardson, the event became the first wide-scale mention of psychedelic drugs to occur in contemporary Western consciousness and it led to a wide interest in the subject.[3] This article also stimulated Timothy Leary to travel to Mexico and make his own investigations. Since then, many others have followed in Wasson's path, and, by 1967, when the psychedelic revolution in the West was in full swing, Maria Sabina had reluctantly become something of a local celebratory, with visitors including Bob Dylan and Mick Jagger, travelling to Mexico to pay their respects. Albert Hofmann also paid his respects and gave her some of Sandoz's psilocybin pills to see what she thought of the synthetic alternative. She admitted that the little yellow pills did indeed appear to contain some of the spirit of the mushroom. But Sabina later came to regret allowing herself to be thrust into the limelight, saying that the foreign visitors, coming in their droves, had ruined the power of her holy sacrament.

Wasson went on to collect many other specimens of different mushrooms and plants such as *salvia divinorum*. It was his specimens that Albert Hofmann used to first identify and synthesise the active psychedelic compound psilocybin. Wasson's continued interest in the subject led to him making claims that mushroom cults were widespread throughout all parts of the world and that the *amanita muscaria* (fly agaric) mushroom was the source of the mysterious Vedic soma — a belief that has been supported by many in the psychedelic community until very recently, though there are now some notable challenges to his ideas.

Mazatec Magic Mushroom Morning Mayhem

There is reliable archaeological evidence that the indigenous people of South and Central America have used psilocybin mushrooms for thousands of years. Mushroom shaped statues and paintings have been discovered in ancient tombs, which supports the view that the use of the mushroom for religious purposes is older than the Spanish conquistadors that tried so hard to eradicate it.

In Guatemala, mushroom-shaped stones have been discovered, which point towards a sacramental use by the ancient Mayans. As I student I travelled with two friends to Guatemala and, after sneaking past the nonchalant pot-smoking guards, we spent the night on the top of the tallest temple of Tikal after everyone else had left. At dawn we had the place to ourselves, looking down from our position above the canopy of the trees. We marvelled as the sky lit up the jungle and surrounded us with coloured birds — only to have our solitude destroyed by a busload of tourists shipped in like a colonial invasion, hoping to be the first people on the temple to enjoy the daybreak after having had a nice night's sleep in their hotels. What they thought when they climbed the steps to find three straggly hippies already there sitting strumming their guitars I do not know.

Psychedelic mushrooms are ubiquitous throughout Central and South America, and were well known to the Aztecs at the time of the Spanish offensive. The ancient pagan practices were viewed as deeply blasphemous and well worth eradicating by the wise and knowledgeable Christians, who lacked the Aztec's understanding of the value of altered states of consciousness as vehicles to communicate with the divine.

In 1656, Dr. Francisco Hernandez had this to say of the hallucinogenic mushrooms: 'When eaten they cause a madness of which the symptom is uncontrollable laughter and all kinds of visions, such as wars and demons'. This grated with the European version of, what I am calling, safely experienced 'spiritual lite', in which the orthodox Christian approach to religion does not allow for followers to actually experience God firsthand. Rather, that privilege is only for the priests, whose job it is to then transmit the message to the flock. In stark contrast, in the shamanic use of the mushroom, the whole community took part in the ritual and directly experienced their gods.

But the practice was not eradicated entirely. It was pushed into secrecy, surviving only in the most remote mountainous parts of the continent. Over time, in certain places Christian beliefs were embraced, adopted and incorporated into the mushroom ceremonies until we begin to see a peculiar crossover between pagan religion and Christianity. And where the practice of spiritual Mexican mushroom use persists today, we still see this hybrid Christian-pagan ceremony. Some of the cults today believe their mushrooms were a gift from the Christian God, and that the mushrooms grew from the earth in the spots where Christ's tears fell as he hung on the cross:

> We wait for our father, we wait for our Father,
> We wait for Christ.
> With calmness, with care,
> Man of breast milk, man of dew,
> Fresh man, tender man,
> And there I give account, the mushroom says,
> Face to face, before Your glory, the mushroom says,
> Yes, Jesus Christ says, there I have an answer.[4]

He Sees When You are Sleeping. He Knows When You're Awake . . .

We will now travel, astrally, from the steamy rainforests of Central America to the frozen wastes of Siberia. During the winter solstice, here we find a fascinating seasonal character, dressed in red with white plumage, a magical being with the power to fly. No, it's not Santa, it's the *amanita muscaria* mushroom. Or are they in fact the same thing?

The role of the *amanita muscaria* mushroom — or 'fly agaric', so called for its amazing capacity, apparently, to scare off flies — has become the classic symbol of psychedelia, folklore and fantasy alike. It is the fat, bright red, spotted white toadstool that appears in children's stories. It also has psychedelic qualities as a result of the active components muscimol and ibotenic acid, which can cause nausea, drowsiness and low blood pressure as a result of its cholinergic effects. Despite its classically lethal appearance, the toxicity, as well as the psychedelic effects of amanita, are not too much to write home about. Certainly, it can cause harm, though reported fatalities are very rare indeed. Furthermore, drying or boiling the mushroom can reduce the toxicity, although the only certain way to avoid being harmed by this or any other vehicle for psychedelic enlightenment is to avoid consuming it.

Use of the *amanita* for spiritual purposes is well known throughout northern Europe, and noted by many scholars, particularly James Arthur, whose book *Mushrooms and Mankind: The Impact of Mushrooms on Human Consciousness and Religion*, is well worth a read.[5] Siberia is particularly famed for it's use of *amanita*. There is a rich shamanistic tradition attached to the use of the mushroom, which still endures today. The Siberian shamans go out in search of their deity dressed in red and white to pay homage to their hunted prize, filling their sacks with the fruits when they find them growing at the base of pine, spruce, fir, birch and cedar trees. Siberian shamans believe these trees point upwards into the heavens, towards the Pole Star, and that eating the flesh of the *amanita muscaria* mushroom is equivalent to scaling the trees to their summit and reaching the sky gods beyond the stars.

Reindeers feature heavily in the lives of these Siberians, which further ties in with the Santa analogies. The reindeer themselves also enjoy spontaneously searching for and eating the spotted mushroom, even drinking each other's or even the human urine of those who have consumed the fruit.[6] Muscimol, the more psychoactive and also the safest of the two active ingredients, is excreted virtually unchanged in the urine and so effective is it at attracting reindeer that Siberian tribesmen will sometimes bottle post-mushroom human or reindeer urine and use it to attract back those beasts that have strayed from the vicinity.

Flying through the sky in a chariot pulled by reindeers, dressed in red, following a star that sits on top of an evergreen tree. It seems that when Coca Cola 'invented' Christmas in their twentieth-century advertising campaign they knew more than a little about the shamans of Siberia.

Objections to the Mushroom Cult

R. Gordon Wasson made much of the Siberian mushroom stories, as well as believing the *amanita muscaria* mushroom was the legendary *soma* of the pre-Hindu texts. He described a rich, worldwide ancient mushroom cult and his ideas gained great popularity in the 1960s. But, more recently, scholars have begun to come up with opposing views. Certainly, in terms of *amanita* being the mythical product *soma*, it seems an unlikely candidate simply because it is not strong enough as a psychedelic drug to produce the kind of mental states described in the *Rig Vedas* — unless (and this is quite possible, of course) those ancient Aryans knew of some tremendous purification techniques which have since been lost in the midst of time.

The British academic Andy Letcher goes a step further to challenge the long-held view (since the sixties) about the widespread use of the magic mushroom in the UK. The sixties gave birth to a myriad of stories about pixies, druids and pagans from these isles, including many theories about the role mushrooms played in the building and worshipping at Stonehenge and other ancient monuments. Despite the wishful thinking of many people, Dr. Letcher argues very persuasively in his book *Shroom* that there is no evidence — either archeologically or, more importantly, *culturally* — to support the idea that magic mushrooms played any part whatsoever in British history until very recently.[7] Even as recently as Victorian times, the mention of liberty caps was very rare, with most mushrooms being understood simply as either edible or poisonous. Some conspiracy theorists would argue that this is because of the Christian anti-psychedelic propaganda of the Middle Ages and beyond to effectively erase such data from the collective knowledge. But, as Letcher says, this has not been the case in South America, where, despite the extreme efforts of the conquistadors, the mushroom cults survived and continued. Letcher's argument about the informal cultural recording of such information is strong. We British are fantastic at preserving our cultural heritage through folk songs and stories, even in the face of powerful political or dogmatic religious forces that try and oppress such traditions. Yet there is no mention of magic mushrooms anywhere in a rich back catalogue of folk songs, drama and art from this country. Nothing, not a single psychedelic sausage. Shakespeare doesn't touch on it and nor does anyone else. This omission just doesn't add up if mushrooms were out there and people were indeed taking them.

On the other hand (and I put this to Letcher when I saw him at our conference last year), how on earth did so many generations of Welsh hill walkers possibly miss the liberty cap mushrooms? It is impossible to walk more than 20 feet across the countryside in November without crushing them underfoot. Dr. Letcher wonders whether in fact the liberty cap mushroom is a relatively recent addition to our natural habitat, relying, as they do, on a particular climate and lots of rich grassland that has only been available in abundance since the seventeenth-century practice of large scale deforestation and farming.[8]

Whenever the mushrooms arrived in Britain, what is certain is that since the sixties it has been very difficult to convince the psychedelic community any other point of view other than one that assumes the whole world revolves around psychedelic drugs.

The Long-standing Use of Peyote Cacti

We now look back across to the other side of the world to meet a small green cactus about which there is no dispute regarding the role it has played in the cultural development of southern Texas and Mexico. The peyote cactus is a slow-growing, spineless green button that peppers the desert scrub. Archaeological finds of the cactus, at least 5000 years old, have confirmed that the native people of America — particularly the Huichol of Mexico — have used this plant as a tool for spiritual worship just as long as any other recorded psychedelic on the planet.[9]

The cactus' active component, mescaline, produces a long-lasting and intensely sustained psychedelic experience accompanied by rich visual phenomena that encourage spiritual searching. It provides a deep connectivity to the earth for those that use it as part of their ceremonial worship, and it is a powerful unifying force for the community. Not only does it cause no demonstrable problems for the community, but recent evidence demonstrates that those tribes that use peyote have better general mental health than those that do not use the cactus. In particular, peyote-using tribes have reduced rates of alcohol dependency, which fits with our knowledge about the important role to be played by psychedelics as psychopharmacological tools to combat addictions. No doubt the anti-alcohol effect is partly attributable to the intense cohesive effect of the traditional cactus-taking ceremonies, which help the native users to resist the tide of Western trappings, of which alcohol is one of the more destructive elements.[10]

As in South and Central America with the traditional pagan use of the psilocybin mushrooms, the peyote ceremonies have also now developed to incorporate aspects of Christian tradition alongside the ancient beliefs. This is exemplified by this quote from Quanah Parker: 'The white man goes into his church and talks about Jesus. The Indian goes into his tepee and talks *with* Jesus.'

Parker, born in 1852, was an important figure in the history of the native American people as he was arguably the most successful to demonstrate an ability to adapt to the changing face of white persecution. For many Native Americans, this means he sold out, but, nevertheless, he remains respected by both sides. Parker was a firm believer in the traditional use of peyote after it was used to heal his wounds when a bull gored him. He was a founder of the Native American Church, which combined Christian and ancient religious elements and kept peyote at the centre of the worship. While mescaline is a Schedule-One controlled substance in the USA and elsewhere, even today Native American members of the church are allowed to legally use peyote as part of their practice (despite the terribly bitter taste).

Ibogaine: Natures Anti-addiction Plant

In the West African countries of the Democratic Republic of Congo and Gabon, many people follow the Bwiti spiritual practice. It is a form of religion in which the root bark of the *tabernanthe iboga* plant is consumed for spiritual purposes.[11] The plant contains the drug ibogaine that produces an intense psychedelic high with an accompanying strong dissociative effect, so users typically report visual hallucinations as well as out of body experiences. This mixed bag of psychoactive effects arises from the complex psychopharmacological profile of ibogaine.

The drug behaves as a partial 5-HT_{2A} agonist — as does LSD, DMT and psilocybin — which explains its classical psychedelic effects. But it also acts to some extent as an NMDA-antagonist (like ketamine) and a kappa-opioid agonist (like *salvia divinorum*), which explains its dissociative effects. The Bwiti incorporates the subsequent extremely dreamlike qualities of the experience into their functional use of the plant.

Used as part of a community ceremony led by an *N'ganga*, who occupies a shamanistic role of priest and respected village elder, the ceremonies have an ostensibly healing purpose in which individuals may seek to communicate with the dead, ask questions of the spirits of ancestors or seek the answers to meaningful personal questions about their health or future. The root bark is chewed or eaten in large quantities and the experience always occurs at night accompanied by elaborate and colourful rituals of drumming, designed to enhance the altered state of consciousness. Many users also experience vomiting and nausea.

The Bwiti use the ibogaine ceremonies as an important rite of passage and it is a hugely significant moment when young men take the plant for the first time. As with other non-Western psychedelic shamanistic ceremonies, in many Bwiti tribes there is a mixture of Christian and more archaic spiritual practice woven into the ceremony.

What makes ibogaine stand out as a therapeutic tool, one that has attracted the attention of the West, is its capacity for treating addictions. It is uncertain how long the West Africans have been using ibogaine as a sacramental tool for their religious purposes, but the anti-addiction qualities have been known to the Western world for around 150 years. The drug appears to be effective at not only relieving the subjective unpleasant effects of withdrawal from dependent drugs such as alcohol and opiates, but also for producing a reduction in long-term craving and reducing habitual, repetitive and obsessional behaviours that often accompany substance dependence. There is good anecdotal and epidemiological evidence for this, supported by the low rates of alcohol dependence by the Bwiti tribe people. Formal clinical trials are underway and will be described in the next chapter.

It is clear that using ibogaine has been of tremendous importance in improving and sustaining community cohesion for the Bwiti. Its use has been credited as having helped Gabon and the Democratic Republic of Congo resist external Western influences such as widespread drug and alcohol use and consumerism. This has got to be a good thing, if only we in the West could recognise it.

The Eerie Effects of the Diviner's Sage: *Salvia Divinorum*

Those who know this plant always refer to it in the female form, so I forgive me while I pay the plant the same respect. She grows in the forests of Oaxaca, Mexico, where she has been used for thousands of years by the Mazatec people as a tool for spiritual worship and still is today.[12]

She exerts her effects via the compound salvinorin A, a potent kappa-opioid agonist, that, like ibogaine, causes dissociative states of altered consciousness. She is very low in physiological toxicity and very high amounts can be consumed. In her native country of use, she is almost always eaten or drunk, either by making a tea from the crushed and infused leaves (about 50 are required) or chewed in great rolled up bundles of leaves like a massive green cigar such that the psychoactive effects come on slowly and build insidiously over time. But when consumed in the West (bought most often by teenage hedonists on the internet), kids usually choose to smoke a purified extract of the plant through a bong, which produces an immediate and intense high and would quite possibly infuriate the natives of Oaxaca if they saw such a practice.

Salvia is held in very high esteem by the Mazatec shamans, who believe she is an incarnation of the Virgin Mary (more of that ubiquitous Christian influence creeping in here). The psychoactive effect is often very trance-like. Some describe it as eerie or spooky, with peculiar visual distortions. She is used in order to produce a visionary state which may be useful for healing of specific ailments or as a tool to help the user gain a greater insight into whatever personal questions they choose to ask her when they start on their journey to the realms of insight opened up by consuming the plant.

A particularly well-known effect is the graceful afterglow that users experience after the more intense psychedelic effects have worn off, which has lead some researchers to postulate whether salvia might have uses as an antidepressant — a clinical application that has also been explored for the dissociative psychedelic ketamine. More about this in coming chapters.

The Sacred Vine: Ayahuasca

Interest in this mysterious South American brew has grown exponentially like a jungle vine in recent years. It now represents a major subject of study for entire university anthropology departments throughout the world. It encompasses elements from chemistry, shamanism, sociology, ecology and legality issues. At our Breaking Convention psychedelic research conference in 2011, we dedicated an entire day's parallel track presentations to the subject. All the talks were packed to the rafters such was the demand amongst the delegates to learn more about this vine. We will have to dedicate even more time to the subject in our 2013 conference.

But What is It All About?

Ayahuasca (which means variously 'vine of the soul' or 'vine of the spirit') is the name for a psychedelic brew made from a number of key ingredients, the main being at least one plant containing DMT and at least one plant containing the essential monoamine oxidase inhibitors (MAOI) required to allow for the DMT to become psychoactive when consumed orally.[13]

Usually the MAOI plant is that of the *banisteriopsis caapi* vine, which contains, among other chemicals, harmine and harmaline. And the DMT commonly comes from the *psychotria viridis* (or chacruna) plant, although a number of alternative plant sources of DMT may be used, including *diplopterys cabrerana* (or chaliponga).

Traditionally, the plants are chopped and ground then boiled together by a shaman with intimate knowledge of the local jungle flora. There is wide variation in the exact ingredients. The leaves, flowers and bark of many other plants may be added to the brew, each with their own idiosyncratic and purposeful intent to provide particular effects. Contemporary scientists marvel at how the traditional shaman could have possibly known which of the many thousands of species of plants combine together to produce the specific desired effects of the brew. In truth, however, there are many such revelations arising from traditional cultures that could teach us in the West a lot, if only we could open our eyes to the fact that just because it does not come from 'big pharma' doesn't mean it isn't important.

Ayahuasca is produced throughout the Amazonian basin in Columbia, Peru and Brazil, and in recent years there has been a significant industry of tourism to these countries for those soul-searching psychonauts inclined to taste its glories in the natural habitat. There are passionate opinions on both sides of the debate about whether such drug tourism is a good or bad thing.

The Ceremony

Ayahuasca is traditionally taken as part of a religious ceremony. The rite is lead by the shaman, who sings songs periodically to enhance and guide the travellers on their inner journeys during which the consumer will engage with aspects of their personal, collective and communal spiritual awareness and pass through different dimensions of a spiritual reality. The intensity of the psychedelic experience is described by many as 'simply colossal', something that is no doubt influenced enormously by the set and setting engendered by a necessary visit to a strange foreign country and a trek through the rainforest to where it takes place.

Ceremonies often involve several separate sittings, in which the drug is taken over the course of many days, and they also incorporate many non-drug rituals as part of the process. There is a strong element of purging — both mentally and physically — and users almost always spend many hours vomiting or passing diarrhoea in the early stages of the intoxication with the drug, all of which contributes to the overall intensity of the experience.

Participants will frequently encounter entities (a phenomenon also seen when DMT is taken artificially in the West) often in the form of jungle animals representing spiritual ancestors, who provide messages and instructions for the journeyer.

Ayahuasca Through the Ages

Ayahuasca was first brought to the attention of the Western world in the 1950s by the explorer and botanist Richard Evan Shultes, who is also credited as being the father of modern ethnobotany for his adventures with psychedelic plants and fungi amongst indigenous populations of the world.

It is thought that the traditional practice of ayahuasca ceremonies amongst Amazonians has been taking place for thousands of years. It was certainly known to the conquistadors of the sixteenth century who dismissed and tried to eradicate the practice, believing the excited psychedelic states induced by the brew were akin to fornicating with the devil, such was the wisdom of those culturally-pure Catholic liberators of old.

William S. Burroughs famously travelled to South America in the 1950s in search of the plant, immortalised in *The Yage Letters*[14] Similarly, it was the search for the magical properties of the sacred vine that set Terence McKenna on his pathway to psychedelic notoriety in the mid 1970s when he tracked through the jungle with his brother Dennis, resulting in his book *True Hallucinations.*[15] In this book, he describes how his South American experience with ayahuasca and psilocybin mushrooms led him to discover his 'novelty theory', which holds that many connected strands of the universe converge together towards an epoch 'eventually reaching a singularity of infinite complexity on the winter solstice in 2012, at which point anything and everything imaginable will occur simultaneously'.

So there's something to look out for while reading this book! Modern living is certainly complex — infinitely so, arguably — but whether it is any more infinite (whatever that means) than at any other time will remain to be seen. I suppose all will be revealed to us on 21st December 2012. In the meantime, we are to sit back passively and wait. How convenient for those who broadcast such things.

Ayahuasca in Modern Times

With the growth of interest in ayahuasca in the West, many people are now seeking the experience. This commonly occurs once we Westerners have latched on to the idea that there is yet another drug out there worthy of exploring, such is the righteous boredom with our modern TV living. And as with the Native American church's claim to use peyote in their ceremonies as an example of the right for religious freedom, a number of ayahuasca-using churches have sprung up making similar claims — the two most prominent being the Brazilian Santo Daime church and the União do Vegetal (UDV). Both these churches have developed worldwide interest and have been subject to legal battles with authorities.

Indeed, the legal status of ayahuasca has become an interesting subject all of its own. DMT itself, in its pure form, is universally accepted as a Class A and Schedule One substance. But, like the debate that continues to rage about psilocybin mushrooms, there remains considerable lack of clarity about whether plants that contain DMT are themselves illegal. After all, if they are that makes the waterways of the UK hotbeds of illegal drug cultivation, as reed canary grass and the gardeners favourite ribbon grass both contain high concentrations of DMT, as do the brains of many mammals (including humans). In short, the concept that vessels that contain DMT can be outlawed is surreally self-defeating. Nevertheless, the law generally stands that, as with mushrooms, as soon as one makes efforts to prepare the DMT-containing plants in someway — for example, by drying or boiling them — one is seen to be heading towards a particular interest in DMT, and one gets busted.

In the UK, we recently had a very sad situation in which a modern-day shaman from the west of England, Peter Aziz, was jailed for possessing and supplying DMT. He was offering ayahuasca to his clients as part of his a well-established

35-year practice and got caught foul of the law when importing plant products from South America. Inevitably, the authorities (and the media) took issue with his atypical (meaning non industry-sanctioned) approach to pharmacology. Many others, myself included, wrote in his support at the time, but to no avail.[16] His legal defence was that of religious freedom, but this rarely satisfies the judge. It seems Christianity's cultural devouring of all in its path is not a phenomenon confined only to the sixteenth century.

The Weed: The Risks, Benefits, Chemistry and Culture of Cannabis

Let us now move from ayahuasca and on to another popular substance: cannabis. This subject is vast and generally beyond the scope of this book. It encompasses so many strands of human developmental culture, from science and sociology to botany, law and medicine, that I will not begin to approach it here. There are so many other books I could recommend for the interested reader, but probably the best of the contemporary tomes on the subject of the green stuff is Julie Holland's *Pot.*[17] Holland is a learned and wise researcher of all things psychedelic, but particularly cannabis and MDMA (she also edited a great book called *Ecstasy: The Complete Guide* a few years ago).[18]

But is cannabis a psychedelic drug? My answer, of course, is yes. Used at low doses the high is far slighter than drugs like LSD or DMT, but at high doses — as one tends to see with the many hydroponic strains of cannabis that most people in the West now smoke — the effects are extremely strong and bordering on the same mental states induced by the classical psychedelics. Our knowledge of the medicinal uses for cannabis continues to grow every year. As with research on compounds like LSD and MDMA, research into cannabis has been difficult because of restrictions on its use by doctors and scientists, although this has begun to shift slightly in recent years. Much of the research on it's potential use in psychiatry revolves around the different constitutional chemicals found in the cannabis plant. There are many hundreds of active components in cannabis but two in particular stand out as important. The first is delta-9 tetrahydrocanibinol, or THC, and the second is cannabidiol, or CBD. THC is generally considered to be the principal chemical that produces the psychoactive, more psychedelic, alerting and trippy effect of the high; and the CBD is the chemical that produces the more relaxed, bodily dreamy effect.

In the field of psychiatry, THC is generally thought to be a psychotomimetic and psychotogenic drug, that is, it can induce psychosis in people who have a genetic predisposition to the condition and it ought to be avoided by those people with schizophrenia. I can say this with relative authority as I, like all psychiatrists, have seen my schizophrenic patients coming back into hospital as a direct result of relapse secondary to heavy cannabis use. This does not mean that I believe cannabis can *cause* schizophrenia in people who don't have that genetic predisposition — if that were the case then we would see a great many more cases of schizophrenia than we do. After all, around 40% of the population smokes the drug and rates of enduring psychosis (schizophrenia) have remained relatively stable at around 1% all over the world since records began. So cannabis does not cause the condition to arise *de novo*, but it can certainly trigger an episode in those who already have it. In such cases, the most likely cause of the psychotic effects is the THC content of the plant.

The cannabidiol on the other hand is another story. There is a general acceptance that CBD may have an antipsychotic effect.[19] Its presence in the natural form of cannabis (not the hydroponically grown skunk weed, which is abnormally high in THC and low in CBD, but the pure grass as grows in the ground of those countries where it is a native species) acts to balance the psychedelic effects of the THC and provide a calming effect. There are many researchers investigating whether CBD in its pure form can act as an antidepressant, an antipsychotic or an anxiolytic drug. This is an area that deserves a great deal more research. In the meantime, as a psychiatrist, and this is what I tell my patients who have decided to continue to smoke, I would say avoid skunk and move on to unadulterated weed or low grade hashish, which would naturally have a higher CBD content, provide a more balanced smoke and also have possible positive neuro-protective factors. But, as mentioned, if there is any personal or family history of psychosis it is best to avoid this drug altogether.

I am all-too-rapidly summarizing a vast amount of research and knowledge here, so do forgive me. Nevertheless, we shall briefly consider a few other aspects of cannabis in it's context as a non-Western contemporary religious sacrament.

Indian Cannabis

Where does cannabis grow? The simply answer to this is that cannabis grows just about anywhere on the planet. It is one of the most hardy plants we know, which is why in the form of hemp it makes such good rope — and canvas, of course. But it thrives best from a psychoactive point of view in the hottest climates, such as Malawi where I went for my medical elective. It also thrives throughout Asia: Thailand, Cambodia, India, Afghanistan, Pakistan, Nepal, Tibet, Mongolia, China, and so forth.

It is well known that the ancient Chinese shamans used cannabis as a vehicle to communicate with the other worlds, and its use by the Greek, Roman and Norse societies is also well documented. But it was particularly central to the development of the Indian culture. The four-thousand-year-old Vedas describe the Hindus use of cannabis very clearly, unlike the more vague descriptions of *soma*. Cannabis was a 'food of the gods' and was venerated by the early Sikhs as a powerful ally in battle. Like the Chinese, who documented the medicinal properties of the plant meticulously, cannabis has always played its part both as a healer of the sick in this world and as a sacramental substance for religious purposes.

Modern Hindu holy men, *sadhus*, still take their cannabis traditionally in the form of *charas* — a handmade resin, sometimes mixed with datura leaves, which they smoke in a tall clay pipe called a chillum. Their presence all over India is abundant. Millions of people chose this lifestyle, that of a solitary wandering monk without possessions or home on the final leg of the Hindu journey towards *moksha* (liberation). One cannot turn a corner in India without seeing one of these old men (and sometimes women) adorned usually in rags, their skin smeared in white ash, contorted in impossible yoga poses and smoking a tall chillum. Smoking cannabis is a sign of devotion to Shiva for these Hindu holy people as they wander barefoot through their magnificent country from one holy site to another on their final pilgrimage (they get free travel on buses and trains), which ends at the banks of the Ganges in Varanasi. Their final opportunity to break the chain of reincarnation, if they haven't achieved *moksha* through their lifetime of devotion, is to be burned in a funeral pyre and floated down the river. India is truly a country out of this world. I can highly recommend a long visit with no set date or ticket for return.

East African and Jamaican Rastafarianism and Cannabis

The Rastafarian way of life arose in Jamaica in the 1930s but has its roots in East Africa and particularly Ethiopia. The Jamaican political activist Marcus Garvey did much to propagate the cohesion of Jamaican fervour for collective organisation and is venerated by the Rastafarian religion, as is the late Emperor of Ethiopia, Haile Selassie I, whose previous name before becoming royalty, Ras Tafari, after which the movement was named.[20]

The hair is traditionally worn long in dreadlocks, and smoking cannabis is a powerful way of demonstrating dedication to god, or *Jah*. Cannabis is central to the life of Rastafarians, who are found all over the world. (When I was on travels in Kenya as a student there was a Rastafarian funeral taking place in which hundreds of devotees followed the procession and gathered at the graveside to smoke copious amounts of cannabis before throwing an eternity's supply of joints and growing plants into the grave for their brother to use in the afterlife's appreciation of Jah.)

Like other psychedelic drug ceremonies mentioned earlier, there is a mixture of Christianity and traditional African religions in Rastafarianism. Parts of the Bible are quoted to validate the spiritual acts of smoking cannabis:

Genesis: 3:18 'Thou shalt eat the herb of the field.'
Proverbs: 15:17 'Better is a dinner of herb where love is, than a stalled ox and hatred therewith.'

The Killer Weed is Here to Stay

With whatever lens one chooses to look at the influence of cannabis through the years, there is no getting away from it's universally abundant presence. It always has been, and probably always will be, the gateway drug of choice for generations of young people. This is not because it has some unique pharmacological trait that makes it lead on to harder things (as the politicians who wish to maintain it's prohibition may tell us) but, rather, because it carries the mantle of being such a mild, safe and harmless prohibited substance, it's very prohibition naturally makes questioning teenagers ask: 'What's so bad about this stuff? The government made out that of if I smoked this I'd be out murdering my granny next week in order to sell her wedding ring for my next fix. What a load of rubbish! I've been lied to. Well, if they are lying about cannabis then they are probably lying about ecstasy and cocaine . . . and heroin . . . so I may as well try those too!'

This prevalent reaction against current drug laws, which is well documented, is very worrying indeed. If the laws are seen to be so unfit for purpose that they actually *encourage* young people to try harder drugs then surely it is time to review them. There will be more commentary on the issue of the illegalisation of cannabis later in the book.

This is What I tell My Teenage Patients About Cannabis

By far the most dangerous aspect of weed is that it is illegal and to be caught with it can ruin your life. The next most risky element is that it causes a degree of demotivation and apathy — that is, after all, it's *raison d'etre* and why people take it. So forget trying to pass your exams if you're smoking a spliff on the way to school each day. After that, the risks get more serious but then the likelihood of succumbing to them is reduced too. For a small number of people — around 1% — cannabis, like many other drugs, is a poison. That 1% is the same 1% that already have, or may be susceptible to developing, schizophrenia. For these people, it really must be avoided. It is well recognized that cannabis use can trigger a psychotic episode in those unfortunate souls who carry the genetic and environmental risk factors for schizophrenia. The genetic risk factors are unavoidable; simply having a family member with a history of psychosis is all it takes. Environmental risk factors, such as stress induced by relationships, are multifarious and not at all specific to schizophrenia. Drug use is the most important of the non-genetic risk factors.

But does cannabis actually *cause* schizophrenia in people who don't have that pre-existing genetic vulnerability? As mentioned, clearly not, or we would see very high rates of schizophrenia amongst the Jamaicans in Jamaica, the Africans in Africa and the Asians in Asia — not to mention in the West — where cannabis is smoked copiously by large numbers of those populations. (We do, incidentally, see increased rates of schizophrenia in black populations living in cities in the UK and other Western countries, but that is different, and most likely due to the stress of social exclusion, poverty and frank racism — both from the wider community and from the medical profession who misconstrue their idiosyncratic and culturally-bound presentation as psychosis.) Hopefully, in future categorical manuals for psychiatric diagnoses we will include the category 'spiritual emergency', which will allow for certain people to behave in a fashion as befits their culture without having to pathologise them further. In the meantime, we remain restricted to the medical model, with all its shortcomings and gross prejudices.

Being a 'Psychedelic Consultant' for Music Television

In 2008, I was contacted by a producer for MTV who, for insurance purposes I assume, needed a medical doctor to comment on a host of unusual psychedelic drugs that she planned to give to people for a show they were developing. The show was called 'Dirty Sanchez' and entailed a group of young Welsh chaps travelling around the world quaffing various local psychoactive plants. It was, I suppose, a less culturally highbrow version of the Bruce Parry programme *The Tribe* that was quite popular at the time.

From what I knew of Dirty Sanchez (and I'll leave the reader to look up what that name means), the Welsh fellows in question were famed for their brash, gung-ho approach to everything they did. For this reason, I was immediately wary of getting involved. I spent some time speaking to the producer, stressing, in no uncertain terms, that if she were to be taking these presenters to all these hidden, sensitive parts of the world to meet shamans and partake in spiritual ceremonies it is essential that they pay close attention to the local customs and behave in a manner of respectful deference and humility. This does not include doing things like nailing one's scrotum to planks of wood, as I believe they have been known to do in the past.

The producer assured me such safeguards would be firmly in place and provided me with the travel itinerary and local substances she had in mind. So, after first sending her detailed instructions on the importance of set and setting and respecting the power and sanctity of the psychedelic substances, I consulted a load of psychedelic textbooks — especially Stafford's *Psychedelics Encyclopedia*[21] and Hofmann and Schultes *Plants of the Gods*[22] — and compiled lists and recommendations for the participants to take on their journeys. They duly got signed off by their insurance company and went on their way. The following notes were supplied on a whole host of natural substances from around the world.

If in South Africa, One Must Try the Plant *Sceletium*

There are at least two species of this plant: *sceletium tortuosum* and *sceletium expansum*. The plant is also known as *mesembryanthemum* or, in South Africa, it is called *kanna* or *channa*. Hottentots have used it for millennia as a vision-enhancing hallucinogen. It can be consumed by smoking, chewing the fermented leaves or absorbing the powder through the mucous membrane of the mouth. The plant contains the psychoactive alkaloid components mesembrine and mesembrenine.

Both these components *can* induce a psychedelic experience, but the main effects of *kanna* are of a mild simulative intoxication not unlike cocaine, with elevated mood, appetite suppression and increased energy. In much higher doses, it may produce a torpor in which the user enters a prolonged state of sedation.

When taken orally in moderate and controllable doses, this drug ought not present as a major health risk as long as participants have a previous good bill of health. As with any cocaine-like stimulants, this drug must be avoided if participants have any pre-existing cardiac problems. Similarly, because the drug acts like a selective serotonin re-uptake inhibitor (SSRI), it must be avoided if participants are also taking any similar antidepressant medication or particularly any monoamine oxidase inhibitors.

As for all psychoactive drugs, the plant is best consumed in facilitative, safe and relaxed surroundings and be sure that some of the party remain drug-free in order to act as guides.

When in Australia You May Wish to Consider Cane Toad Licking?

Cane toad licking has received considerable media attention in recent years. The active components are 5-MEO-DMT and bufotenin. It is probably more popular in Australia than anywhere else — and the toads are not actually licked, as such. One shudders to think how this peculiar pastime was ever discovered.

The common name of cane toad is derived from the original purpose of using it to eradicate pests in sugar cane crops. There are several species of toads that produce venom that has psychoactive properties. The most popularly used as a drug is *bufo alvarious*, which contains both 5-MeO-DMT and bufotenin. All the other bufo species contain only bufotenin.

The cane toad can grow up to six inches in length, has dry and warty skin, and can be grey, brown, red-brown or olive in colour, with varying patterns. There are distinct ridges above the eyes that run down the snout. Cane toads have a life expectancy of 10 to 15 years in the wild and as long as 20 years in captivity.

The toad produces the venom from the parotid gland behind its ear, which can be gently 'milked' from the gland, dried and smoked (usually in a small glass pipe). The toad then replenishes its store of venom within a month. There is no need to kill the toad to extract the venom. However, sometimes the toad is killed, dried and eaten, smoked or boiled into a foul-tasting tea and drunk. On smoking the venom, the effects may be significantly strong — not unlike that of psilocybin (magic mushrooms) or LSD. The effects come on rapidly and may include distortions in visual perception, profound alterations in thinking and identity and distortions in the perception of time.

There are no mentions of ancient indigenous examples of using cane toad venom as a sacrament. The toads were only introduced to Australia in the twentieth century. However, they have since become popular with Australian hippies.

If You Get to Tonga, You May Want to Check Out the Kava

Kava (*piper methysticum*) is an evergreen shrub with large heart-shaped leaves and woody stems. One can mash up its roots and make a cold drink for intoxicating purposes. Its active ingredients are called kavalactones and are certainly psychoactive. The drink causes effects for up to eight hours, including throat and mouth numbness, nausea and ataxia, which cause a lot of falling over. People report feeling relaxed and having reduced social inhibitions, much like drinking alcohol.

In Pacific Polynesia, where it is most popular, it is usually enjoyed in the evenings at moderate and gentle doses as part of a communal activity. But the MTV producer felt her boys would probably want to snort their kava. I therefore had to warn them that, unless they were using a very concentrated extract, they would most likely need to snort a large amount of the material to get a dose, and doing it repeatedly could definitely lead to serious sinus problems and damage to the nasal passages. There is no historical tradition of snorting kava, so there's no data on the practice. I don't know whether they did end up snorting it or not. Let's hope not — though its probably better than nailing one's scrotum to a plank.

Next Stop India, for Indian Snakeroot

Also called serpentwood or rauwolfia, this is an evergreen shrub found in Indian forests, which, in spring, is peppered with white and pink flowers. The active ingredient is the alkaloid reserpine, which produces a primarily sedative and depressant effect. It is not known to be especially psychedelic but has been used in Ayurvedic medicine for thousands of years to treat everything from poisonous reptile bites to insanity.

Calamus! Calamus! Will You Do the Fandango?

Calamus — also known as sweet flag, sweet sedge, sweet root and myrtle grass — grows in wetlands as leafy stems projecting upwards bearing little yellow-brown flowers. It is the root that is chewed and the taste is horrible — extremely bitter. The active components are alpha and beta-asarone. They increase energy and reduce hunger, like a stimulant, but at the same time also produce a calming sensation. Sweet flag is therefore interesting as both a stimulant and sedative simultaneously. It has been compared by some to LSD; but those familiar with the effects of LSD may disagree.

If You Stop in South East Asia, Be Sure to Ask for Kratom

Kratom has become popular in the West in recent years since the internet took notice. Locally, in South East Asia, it often gets called mambog and can be found all over Thailand, Malay Peninsula, Borneo and New Guinea. One dries the leaves, which are then smoked or chewed. Contained in it, among other indole alkaloids, is the substance mitragenine, which, not unlike calamus, can be simultaneously stimulating, like cocaine, and soothing, like morphine. Interestingly, it has been used as an opium substitute to cure opiate addiction.

Nonda Mushrooms

These mushrooms, from Papua New Guinea, are most interesting for their visual effects as they are famed for causing what psychiatrists call Lilliputian hallucinations in which little people or animals are seen. The mushrooms themselves, *boletus manicus* and *boletus kumeus*, have a 15cm diameter, creamy white cap, and contain various indole alkaloids. Because of the mushroom's propensity to cause violent rages it may be taken by natives before planning to kill another person. Not one for the Glastonbury Festival then.

The 'Rubbish' Pitohui Bird

Also from New Guinea comes the brightly coloured hooded pitohui bird — one of a well-known group of toxic birds, which the locals refer to as 'rubbish' because it is generally no good to eat (unless laboriously skinned and then treated by roasting in charcoal). If the bird pecks or scratches a human, he or she develops a swelling and tingling. The birds produce an endotoxin called homobatrachotoxin that comes from their diet of choresine beetles, as a defence against predators, which are mainly snakes and other birds. The taste is extremely bitter and it almost always makes humans very sick. There are no contemporary reports of it being psychedelic (except to look at, given its incredible plumage) but there are some Aztec documents from the sixteenth century that speak of a bird that induced visions. This could be the pitohui bird, at a stretch.

The Fierce Agara Leaves of Papua New Guinea

The colossal *galbulimima belgraveana* tree, which grows up to 90-feet tall, sports glossy leaves and a grey, scaly bark. When the bark and leaves are boiled together with another plant, *ereriba*, to make a tea, there are over twenty different alkaloids at play that induce a deep slumber during which visions are experienced. A violent tremor is also common, and the people of the Okapa region (where the tree grows) use agara leaves to make men fierce in order to counteract malevolent power that is thought to be the cause of a variety of illnesses.

The Visionary Plants of Africa

Africa is a splendidly mystical place. It oozes with spirituality just as much as the more overt experience of India, but with a far more serene and considered tone. Every rock, tree and river breathes deep, distant spiritual history. My travels there have been more meditative and contemplative than the screeching rancour of the East, but certainly no less spiritual.

The concept of African 'witch doctors' is well known. We Western doctors struggle with the idea of people practicing medicine without the proper evidence-based methods. Time will tell who offers the best therapeutic interventions for full holistic well-being.

Ubulawu is a general term used by the Zulu's to mean visionary plants and there are hundreds of different barks, bulbs, vines, roots, leaves, seeds and flowers which are chopped up and used to make *ubulawu*, a white frothy mixture that is taken orally. Plants incorporated in *ubulawu* include African dream root (or *heimia salicifolia*), *acacia xanthophloea*, *behnia reticulata* and *dianthus mooiensus*. Usually, around two dozen different plant species — often those growing near to rivers — are used when the doctor makes up his or her *ubulawu*. Unlike the South American *ayahuasca*, the effects may be wildly idiosyncratic depending on the preparation of the mixture. Generally, dreams will be enhanced and at times certainly a full-blown psychedelic experience is possible. African shamans used the medicine as a divine tool, as this quote testifies:

> Ubulawu belongs to the ancestors. It opens your brain to work. It is used to induce or clarify dreams of ancestral spirits and opens minds to receive the messages of the ancestors.

When I was in Malawi for two months, working in an obstetric hospital (that's another story), I visited a local witch doctor because I was getting a lot of arthritic pain from my distant childhood fractures. The man was adorned in animal skins and shuffled about fussing over plastic pots, bits of tangled defunct electrical equipment and live animals that wandered in and out of his hut throughout the session. He didn't use any visionary plants (or at least didn't give me any, but could well have been on them himself). Instead, he held my ankle for a long time, murmured a lot, tossed runes and bothered the ashes in the fire creating billowing sparks. When we left I asked my Malawian guide to translate what the man had said about my foot. She smiled and said: 'He says when you die will still have both your legs'. That is a relief to know!

The Zulu's Strawflower Smoke

Strawflower is tall, being of the sunflower family, and it produces clusters of golden-yellow flowers. It grows in Africa, and the Zulu traditionally smoke the dried herb. Although native doctors use it to induce trances the active ingredients, coumarins and diterpenes, are not known to have any psychedelic effects.

Jenkem

When the MTV producer asked me whether it was worth her boys being filmed consuming jenkem I thought, 'yes, but rather them than me'.

Jenkem is allegedly human faecal matter and urine, which have been left to ferment in a bottle and then the gases are collected and inhaled. Presumably, the active ingredients are methane and ethanol and the effect is, supposedly, like a mild version of sniffing glue. On the other hand, some people say that the whole concept of jenkem is a hoax designed to catch out drug tourists. Perfect.

Pandanus Nuts

The plant that produces these heavy fruit is called screw pine and it grows along the coast in salt marshes. Huge quantities of the nuts need to be eaten to get the desired effect, which is not always especially pleasant. Like many of the earth's plants, these nuts contain dimethyltryptamine (DMT), which may cause hallucinations. Pandanus nuts are used in folk medicine, magic and for ceremonial purposes and have been said to cause an outbreak of 'irrational behaviour' called Karuka madness.

What Happened to the Dirty Sanchez Boys?

I don't know exactly what happened to the Dirty Sanchez crew on their trips. The producer never sent me a DVD of the series, as I requested. But one night several years later, I happened to see a program featuring two Welsh boys sitting respectfully in meditative poses with a shaman from somewhere or other. I was impressed to see they were displaying appropriate reverence to the local customs (though they did slunk off after a while when they thought the meditating shaman had fallen asleep). Then, sure enough, at the end credits there I was: 'Psychedelic Consultant — Dr. Ben Sessa'. Job well done.

CHAPTER 8

The Psychedelic Renaissance Part One: Movers and Shakers

The next two chapters will focus on the contemporary research projects and the people behind them that have emerged in the last twenty-five years. For those of us in the field, it is exciting that today's society and medical profession are deciding to look again at the psychedelic compounds. It may be that we missed something important when the research was shelved forty years ago. Who knows how far we may have travelled in the field of psychiatry had we continued to study the psychedelic drugs at the rate they were being explored between 1950 and 1966. The current climate in which far fewer psychoactive drugs dominate our clinical work would look a lot different had we continued to use psychedelics since the 1950s. As it is, the antidepressants, antipsychotics and mood stabilisers remain the clinical profession's psychiatric drugs of choice. We may also have found ourselves further along in our understanding of human consciousness. We have sadly missed out on both possibilities, but now we have a chance to make amends and reintroduce these tools into our clinical armoury again.

A Coming Together of Disparate Tribes

Like all groups who feel somewhat on the fringes of the mainstream, the psychedelic research community has always been good at organising itself into cohesive collectives and affiliations in which like-minded folk can share ideas and disseminate their findings. Their members also tend to be those sorts of people who like writing, feel an urge to organise the minority masses and enjoy staying up late. The result is a lot of words being written and spoken.

Under the auspices of Timothy Leary's *International Federation for Internal Freedom*, the journal *The Psychedelic Review* ran from 1963 to 1971. It started out with a scientific slant, encouraging a melting pot of ethnological, botanical, sociological, medical, psychiatric, cross-cultural and anthropological perspectives to discuss psychedelic drugs. By the end of the sixties, the journal had begun to slightly slant away from the academic focus, and gravitate towards the hippie cultural values predominant at the time. Today, original copies change hands for large amounts of money on eBay, but all the journal's editions are now also available online to read for free.[1]

The Entheogen Review was a similarly targeted quarterly publication. Edited by David Aardvark and K. Trout, it ran from 1992 to 2008, and was host to the best of the old and the new, emerging psychedelic devotees. It is now also available to everyone online at Erowid (see below).

As in all fields of study, the internet has hugely increased the coming together of widely disseminated psychedelic interest groups. This has been particularly important for exploring multinational non-Western perspectives, and has allowed a mixing of medical and popular cultural movements to stay in close contact. There have been some fascinating gatherings, conferences and festivals in recent years in which the boundaries between medicine, art, cross-cultural studies and partying have been blurred, presenting unrivalled opportunities for multi-disciplinary and multi-dimensional learning.

Below are a few of the current groups, conferences, affiliations and websites operating right now that I know of.

Some Important Contemporary Psychedelic Organisations

1. The Multidisciplinary Association for Psychedelic Studies (MAPS)

MAPS is an immensely important psychedelic research organisation, formed in America in 1986 as a result of Rick Doblin's insistence to fight the rushed criminalization of MDMA by the US government. MAPS employs a skilled team of psychedelic researchers and media-savvy event organisation experts. With a clear educational strategy, a code of free access to information and Doblin's inspirationally motivational style at the helm, MAPS reviews papers, sets up, runs, organises and funds clinical and non-clinical research and provides a platform for all aspects of psychedelic happenings all over the world. It also publishes books on psychedelic healing and culture, and maintains an important presence at international conferences and gatherings exploring the subject of psychedelic drugs.[2]

2. The Heffter Research Institute

Founded in 1993 by David Nichols, George Greer, Mark Geyer, Dennis McKenna and Charles Grob, the Heffter Research Institute is named after the German psychopharmacologist who first studied the compound mescaline. With research centres in Los Angeles, New York, Arizona and Baltimore in the US, and at the University of Zurich in Switzerland, the Heffter Institute incorporates an impressive board of high-level clinical and research scientists from around the world. They design and oversee clinical, pre-clinical and socio-cultural research concerning psychedelic drugs and provide education to the medical profession, policy makers and the research community.[3]

3. The Beckley Foundation

Founded in 1998, the brainchild of Amanda Feilding from the UK, the Beckley Foundation operates from beautiful surroundings in rural Oxfordshire. Since its inception, the foundation has been lobbying for changes to international drug law policy. In recent years, there have been increasing collaborations between Beckley and various research projects at Bristol and Imperial universities in the UK, as well as other international projects. Feilding's inimitable personality is matched only by the tireless effort and unswerving personal determination she puts into pushing back the frontiers of consciousness research.[4]

4. Council of Spiritual Practice

This is an organisation convened in 1993 in San Francisco by Bob Jesse. Its mission is to increase people's access to 'direct experience of the sacred'. The council aligns itself with many methods and practices to do this, including psychedelic drug use and meditation. It provides a strong support for the use of entheogens as a vessel through which to connect to a greater sense of cosmic unity. The council supports psychedelic events (it co-hosted the 2011 MAPS conference in San Jose) and is keen to propagate the work of past and present psychedelic studies, particularly those that pertain to the spiritual aspects of the experience.[5]

5. The Gaia Media Foundation

Dieter Hagenbach and Lucius Werthmueller founded Gaia Media in Basel in 1993. In 2006, they hosted the most special of all recent psychedelic conferences, the tremendous 'LSD Conference' in Basel to celebrate the 100th birthday of its illustrious board member, Albert Hofmann. In 2008, a follow-up event was staged: the World Psychedelic Forum. Gaia Media is a forum for artistic expression, constellation of ideas and dissemination of information about many esoteric aspects of science and the arts, including the clinical, spiritual and personal use of psychedelic drugs.[6]

6. Horizons: Perspectives on Psychedelics

Originally set up by Kevin Balktick in 2007 in the wake of the Gaia Media Foundation's hugely popular LSD conference, this New York-based annual conference covers the social, political, clinical and multicultural aspects of psychedelic drugs. Neal Goldsmith, a multitalented speaker, organiser of people and author of *Psychedelic Healing*, curates the annual meetings and holds year-long lecture series gathering minds together.[7]

7. Breaking Convention

This is the UK-based conference that had its first outing in 2011. It was a fabulous group effort organised by the seat of our pants by Dave King, Cameron Adams,

Anna Waldstein, Dave Luke and myself. The summer meeting gathered over 600 delegates and speakers from 29 different countries and a broad range of topics was debated, which reflected the multidisciplinary backgrounds of the organisers. We covered subjects from ethno-cultural-botany and sociology to binaural beats, receptor profiles, clinical innovations and historical accounts of experiential moments in psychedelic history. There were films, bands, flowers, incense, smart drinks and video links to Ram Dass and Stanislav Grof. We plan to repeat the conference in 2013 and hope as many people as possible can get involved and be part of the organisation with us.[8]

8. The Open Foundation

The Open Foundation arose, like New York's Horizons conference, out of the success of the 2006 LSD Conference put on by the Gaia Media Foundation. A Dutch-based group, philosopher Joost Breeksema and anthropologist Dorien Tatalas founded Open. Their mission is to stimulate research, educate and encourage debate on the subject of psychedelic drugs and the psychedelic experience.[9] They held a major international conference in 2010, Mind Altering Science, and plan another for October 2012, to be held in Amsterdam.

9. Erowid

Erowid is an extraordinary online library resource, quite like no other, with detailed information on the pharmacology, history, effects, chemistry, legality, politics and cultural aspects of hundreds of psychoactive substances.[10] The lovingly nurtured creation of Fire and Earth Erowid, it is an impressive piece of technology. There is more on this website than one can read in a lifetime, with a dynamic emergence of users' trip reports and the latest breaking news about every known drug, new and old. The Erowid crew is also a popular presence at the major psychedelic gatherings and conferences, dishing out their unbiased and measured important advice for psychonauts, drug-geeks and naïve learners everywhere.

10. Bluelight

This is a Dutch-based online resource for psychedelic drug users all over the world to share their experiences about drugs, doses, developments and happenings. Thousands of posts are collected, moderated and disseminated by a crew of active psychonauts with a keen eye on latest developments. They pride themselves on providing freely available information to all drug users as a means of reducing the harm caused by careless and misinformed use of drugs. There is a particular focus on MDMA/ecstasy use, and resources include information about pill testing, and education and careers advice as well as access to the artistic and musical worlds connected with the psychedelic experience.[11]

11. Shroom With a View

Formed in 2009, this is a slickly designed online forum specialising in regular podcast broadcasts providing wide coverage of the psychedelic community. Particular attention is given to the psilocybin mushroom experience. Shroom regularly interviews characters from the psychedelic community and also has a great online bookshop.[12]

12. Neurosoup

Founded and hosted by the ever popular Krystal Cole, this website provides an exhaustive flow of regular video clips and podcasts in which Cole interviews users and experts, and describes experiences with just about every psychedelic drug imaginable.[13] Her site provides useful insights and education for psychedelic voyagers, with a strong emphasis on harm reduction, assistance for addictions and encouragement of careful use. In 2006, I had the pleasure of contributing a chapter to her *Neurosoup* book.[14]

13. Reality Sandwich

This is a beautifully conceived online resource for many aspects of ecology, consciousness expansion, art, music, protest and shamanistic openings, with a particular emphasis on psychedelics. As it says on Reality Sandwich's website: 'Evolving consciousness, bite by bite'.[15]

14. Regeneration

With its first outing due in summer 2012 the Regeneration Festival is the invention of David Dyerson of the splendid psychedelic light show *Bardo Lights*. An offshoot arising from Breaking Convention 2011, those of us involved wholly support Dyerson and his vision to bring a taste of multimedia psychedelic experience to the fields and hedgerows of Surrey. Let's hope there will be more light from Regeneration in the future.[16]

15. Psychedelic Spirituality Forum

Psychedelic Spirituality Forum is one of the newest educational organisations that chose to spread mostly through social networks such as Facebook. The idea behind it was to reach young people and encourage them to freely participate in any beneficial activity linked to psychedelics. The structure promotes the ideas of safety and scientific knowledge, ancient wisdom and spiritual aspects of psychedelic drugs. The organisation has spread informative paper leaflets about psychedelic therapies (such as ibogaine), given out t-shirts, helped in organising screenings of documentaries about psychedelics sacraments.[17]

16. Students For Sensible Drug Policy

An American organisation founded in 1998 by and for students all over the world, the SSDP is primarily concerned with campaigning for a more fit-for-purpose, evidence-based approach to the international drug laws. It fights against the War on Drugs, based on the clear understanding that the War on Drugs is harming, not protecting, young people from the physical, societal and legal dangers of drug abuse.[18]

Some Important Contemporary Psychedelic Researchers[19]

There are many people worldwide who have contributed significantly to the renaissance of clinical, anthropological and social psychedelic research. There are, of course, many more from the old guard of Huxley, McKenna, Hofmann, Osmond, Leary, and so forth who have since departed their mortal forms and will not be found on this list below. And there are also lots from the last generation, who started their work in the 1950s, 1960s and 1970s and are still producing valuable contributions to the field today, such as Metzner, Grof, Weil, Shulgin, Stolaroff, Greer, Fadiman, Richards and Ram Dass. The ones mentioned here are those slightly newer additions (at least in terms of when they started publishing), whose contributions to research in recent years has spearheaded a new generation of interest in the psychedelic compounds in order that new young researchers can be inspired to take up the mantle and enter the field.

Cameron Adams is a medical and ecological anthropologist from Arizona with an interest in psychedelic medicine and ecological consciousness. Until recently, he was a lecturer at the University of Kent where he was conducting web-based research on virtual communities. In 2011, he co-founded and co-chaired the UK's Breaking Convention conference and now is the chief editor of Breaking Convention Publications.

Susan Blackmore is a psychologist with a special interest in memetics (the study of memes) and has contributed widely to this field. She is also a well-known broadcaster in the UK and never shies of supporting broad-minded and progressive research. She has a degree in parapsychology and has spoken out vociferously in support of psychedelic research.

Robin Carhart-Harris is a psychopharmacologist from the UK, with an unusual training in rather separate fields. His dual degrees in psychoanalysis and psychopharmacology have prepared him perfectly to be the person to explore the neural apparatus with a keen eye on both physiology and the psychology of its function. Having met him in Basel in 2006 and then worked beside him in Bristol University psychopharmacology department, we have become close friends. Carhart-Harris's contributions to psychedelic research in this country have been prolific from the beginning. His recent work with psilocybin is giving the field of neuroscience plenty to think about. He now works at Imperial University, London, and there is certainly far more to come from him.

Valerie Curran is Professor of Psychopharmacology at University College London, where she specialises in research that links our understanding of how drugs work at a neurotransmitter level with how they are producing particular subjective psychological and cognitive effects. During her career she has carried out important work with cannabis, ketamine and MDMA. And as clinical lead in her local NHS Substance Misuse Service, she is keen to see that her research accurately reflects the risk and safety profiles of the psychedelic drugs. In this respect, she has contributed valuably to the evidence-based argument about the relative safety of MDMA-assisted psychotherapy.

Alicia Danforth is a clinical and transpersonal psychologist from the States. She has had an impressive start to her psychedelic career and also has an assured future ahead of her in the field. She assisted Charles Grob in his Harbor-UCLA cancer-anxiety psilocybin study and her current research is looking at whether there can be a role for MDMA in managing autism.

Paul Devereux is a UK-based commentator on anthropology and archaeology and a Fellow with the International Consciousness Research Laboratories (ICRL) group at Princeton University, USA. He has a special interest in the role psychedelics have played in the development of human culture and also speaks, broadcasts and writes on a wide range of esoteric subjects including UFOs, ley lines and dowsing.

Rick Doblin studied psychology and policy studies and founded the Multidisciplinary Association of Psychedelic Studies in 1986, which he continues to direct. He remains at the forefront of psychedelic research as a popular figure inspiring new generations of young psychedelic researchers all over the world.

Amanda Feilding is the founder and director of the Beckley Foundation. Her own history is one so colourful and fabulous it would take an entire book to cover it. Since her exposure to the embryonic psychedelic awakenings in London in the early 1960s, her trepanning, her long friendship with Albert Hofmann and her current close associations with contemporary researchers all over the world, Amanda has seen it all. She continues to push the boundaries of consciousness research as a brave enthusiast looking in with great interest to the decidedly technical world of high-level psychopharmacology research.

Friederike Fischer is a medical doctor from Germany who became a psychotherapist in Switzerland. Together with her husband Konrad, she has contributed enormously to contemporary psychedelic research, though in a slightly unconventional manner. Trained as part of the psycholytic study group that formed legally in Switzerland between 1988 and 1993 (which also provided training for other psychedelic researchers Peter Oehen and Peter Gasser), Friederike went on to provide several years of underground psychedelic therapy to a number of patients using LSD, MDMA and 2C-B, developing an effective technique to work constructively with these substances, which can inform research and clinical work to come.[20]

Robert Forte is a professor at the California Institute of Integral Studies. Having worked with both Mircea Eliade and Stanislav Grof, his qualifications for understanding the role of psychedelics and society are considerable. He is the editor of several recent important books on psychedelics: *Entheogens and the Future of Religion, Outside Looking In* (about Timothy Leary) and *The Road To Eleusis: Unveiling the Secret of the Mysteries*, by Wasson, Hofmann and Ruck. Robert has a deep and influential interest in the power of entheogens to inform our social, spiritual, creative and athletic development; including some interesting ideas about how magic mushrooms can improve our understanding and mastery of golf.

Peter Gasser is a Swiss psychiatrist with prior training in psychedelic psychotherapy during the brief window of psychedelic activity that occurred in Switzerland between 1988 and 1993. He is currently carrying out the first and only contemporary LSD psychotherapy study underway anywhere in the world.

Mark Geyer is one of the co-founders of the Heffter Research Institute and contributes to work carried out at the Heffter's research facility based at Zurich University. He specialises in translational research and looks at the links between the behavioural effects of psychedelic drugs and cognitive processing in humans and animals.

Neal Goldsmith is a psychotherapist from New York and the author of a recent book *Psychedelic Healing*. He is the curator of New York's Horizons psychedelic conference. His clinical practice incorporates elements of transpersonal, humanistic and Eastern traditions and is particularly useful for adults undergoing existential crises or couples coping with significant changes in their lives. His gentle and persuasive approach to the study of psychedelic drugs and people in general as healing agents is an inspiration to all.

Roland Griffiths is Professor of Behavioral Biology and Neuroscience at Johns Hopkins University School of Medicine. As a doctor with an interest in alcoholism and psychopharmacology, he consults for innumerable organizations and institutions worldwide, and has been publishing in the academic field since 1969. But it his recent work with psilocybin that has attracted enormous attention from the psychedelic community. Having explored, in 2006, psilocybin's ability to produce spontaneous spiritual experiences, he is now going on to determine the extent to which the drug can produce lasting positive personality changes and how this might be applied to two fields of psychiatry that are notoriously difficult to treat: addictions and personality disorders.

Charles Grob is a professor of Child and Adolescent Psychiatry at UCLA and on the board of the Heffter Research Institute. He has contributed widely to psychedelic research in recent years with his study exploring the role for psilocybin as a tool to manage the anxiety and existential issues associated with end-stage cancer. His professional position as a child psychiatrist provides particular inspiration for me to help juggle my own clinical and research roles.

John Halpern is an Assistant Professor of Psychiatry at McLean Hospital Harvard Medical School. His research projects since the mid 1990s have included looking at cognitive functioning of MDMA and ayahuasca users, the use of psilocybin and LSD to relieve cluster headaches and the Native American Church use of peyote. He started a clinical project examining the use of MDMA as an agent to treat anxiety in patients with end-stage cancer but this was shut down because of participant enrolment difficulties. He continues to play an important role in psychedelic research.

Graham Hancock is a UK-based sociology writer and researcher of many unusual aspects of human history. His interests include ancient civilisations, myths and legends and the role for altered states of consciousness in the evolution of human consciousness.

Julie Holland is a New York psychiatrist with extensive experience working at Belleview Hospital (and author of *Weekends at Bellevue*).[21] She has an impressive curriculum vitae, spanning all aspects of the renaissance of psychedelic research. She has edited major works on MDMA and cannabis, and continues to broadcast on the importance of recognising the relative risks and safety of psychedelic drugs as tools for medical, personal and societal development.

David King is an anthropologist from the University of Kent, UK, with a special interest in the medical uses of psychedelic plants and fungi in the development of human culture. As co-founder, King has been instrumental in the origins and maintenance of the UK's Breaking Convention conference and also worked at the Beckley Foundation. He currently resides in Singapore where he is attempting to explore drug policy in what is one of the harshest environments on the planet for this field of research.

Evgeny Krupitsky is a psychiatrist from St. Petersburg, Russia with a special interest in addictions. Inspired by the work of Osmond with LSD in the 1950s, Krupitsky lead the world in ketamine psychotherapy research in the

1990s, applying this substance to treatments for alcohol and opiate dependence. He used the depth and powerful influence of the ketamine psychedelic experience alongside individual and group psychotherapy to achieve impressive abstinence results in chronic substance mis-users.

Andy Letcher is a UK-based folk activist and writer. His 2007 book, *Shroom,* has opened an interesting debate about the extent (or not) to which magic mushrooms have played an important part in shaping the culture of Britain.[22] He is a prolific writer on the subject of folk culture (and also plays an impressive number of traditional instruments).

David Luke is a UK-based academic psychologist, Senior Lecturer at Greenwich University, London where he teaches an undergraduate course on the psychology of exceptional human experiences. He is also president of the Parapsychological Association and a past research associate at the Beckley Foundation. He chairs the Ecology, Cosmos and Consciousness lecture series at the October Gallery in Bloomsbury, London and has a special interest in altered states of consciousness and paranormal phenomena.

Louis Eduardo Luna studied comparative religion at Stockholm University and now works and writes extensively on the subject of shamanism, particularly as it pertains to South American culture. He has published books on ayahuasca and is Director of the Research Center for the Study of Psychointegrator Plants, Visionary Art and Consciousness in Florianópolis, Brazil.

Dennis McKenna is the brother of Terence. Their lives have been woven together through years of shared research and travel in both its the planetary and intra-planetary forms. Dennis, a botanist by training, is no less a force in academic psychedelic research than his brother. He is a highly respected orator on ayahuasca, sits on the board of directors at the Heffter Research Institute and continues to contribute widely to the field.

Michael Mithoefer is a psychiatrist from Charleston University, South Carolina, with a life-long special interest in PTSD and psychedelic therapy. His research led him to meet Rick Doblin in 2000, which began their relationship to instigate the world's first randomised, controlled, double-blind clinical study with MDMA, published in 2010. Mithoefer continues to work closely with MAPS, currently running further trials with MDMA-assisted psychotherapy and, together with his wife Annie, a registered nurse and co-therapist on the MDMA studies, they offer training for future MDMA therapists throughout the world.

David Nichols is Professor of Medicinal Chemistry and Pharmacology at Purdue University, USA. He is the co-founder and director of the Heffter Research Institute. He has contributed numerous works to the pre-clinical study of psychedelic drugs and acts as consultant to NIH, NIMH and NIDA advisory groups. He is a Fellow of the Academy of Pharmaceutical Sciences and American Association of Pharmaceutical Scientists. He gives great lectures that render the mysterious worlds of chemistry and neurotransmitters accessible to all.

David Nutt is a British psychiatrist and one of the UK's leading neuropsychopharmacologists, having held senior positions at the British Association of Psychopharmacology and the Presidency of the European College of Neuropsyhcopharmacology. He specialises in addiction, anxiety and sleep disorders. Until 2009, he headed-up the psychopharmacology department at Bristol University and now holds the post of Edmond J. Safra Chair in Neuropsyhcopharmacology at Imperial College, London. In recent years, he has become well known through his courage to speak out in favour of his patients against what he sees as biased government interference in medical research. He is an enthusiastic critic of the current drug laws, which he feels have limited evidence-based validity and are no longer fit for purpose. He runs a vibrant research department and is always keen to nurture new talent and fresh ideas.

Andy Parrot is a British psychologist and psychopharmacologist working at Swansea University. He has contributed a plethora of papers looking at some of the sub-clinical changes occurring in groups of ecstasy users. Parrot deserves accolade for publishing one of the few studies in which the majority of subjects experienced a predominantly negative affect under the influence of MDMA.[23] His views on the acute and chronic dangers of ecstasy use, while not contributing meaningfully to the risk-benefit argument that is central to any clinical approach for a potential new medicine, have made for some interesting debates between us over the years, which I hope will continue.

Torsten Passie is Assistant Professor for Consciousness Studies at Hannover Medical School in Germany. For more than twenty years he has studied psychedelic drugs, altered states of consciousness and clinical shamanic practices. He has worked with Hanscarl Leuner, a leading authority on psychedelic drugs and carried out research with cannabis, ketamine, nitrous oxide, and psilocybin. In 2011, he published a detailed account of the psychopharmacology of LSD.[24]

Daniel Pinchbeck is one of many professional psychonauts, meticulously recording his journeys through the psychedelic landscapes, mapping the inner cosmos as he experiments with new mental states and beats the path providing cartography for others to follow. More about experiential journeying than science, his popular works emphasise the vanity of separating these concepts at all when it comes to psychedelic drugs.

George Ricaurte found fame in the world of psychedelic research for his publication of a severely flawed study in 2002 that suggested there was neurotoxicity in primates given moderate doses of MDMA.[25] However, due to a mix up with the labels (in his laboratory or elsewhere, the exact truth is not known) the animals never actually received MDMA but rather the toxic compound methamphetamine. Ricaurte subsequently suffered the humiliation and damage of a retraction of his article from the journal *Science*, but not before it had done untold damage to the image of MDMA research.[26]

Andy Roberts is an UK-based attractively wizened writer and investigator of all things mysterious and offbeat. A lover of nature, psychedelic music and folk history, in 2008 he published an important book, *Albion Dreaming: A Popular History of LSD in Britain*, and continues to provide insights into the role psychedelics have played in shaping this nation and humankind in general.[27]

Thomas Roberts is a professor at the Department of Leadership, Educational Psychology and Foundations at Northern Illinois University, USA. He has had a long history studying the psychedelic drugs and their impact on the development of the human species. He has been teaching his students about this subject since the 1980s and is also author of the wonderfully futuristic and enthusiastic book *Psychedelic Horizons*.[28]

Andrew Sewell is a USA-based psychiatrist and neurologist working at Harvard Medical School. He has been particularly interested in the role psychedelic plants, fungal alkaloids and LSD might have for alleviating cluster headaches and, together with John Halpern, has been looking in to developing a study to investigate this phenomenon.[29]

Rick Strassman is Clinical Associate Professor of Psychiatry at the University of New Mexico School of Medicine and also president and co-founder of the Cottonwood Research Foundation, which is dedicated to consciousness research. In 1995, he published the first human psychedelic research study in modern times, opening up the way for the resurgence of work since, when he studied the subjective psychological effects of DMT on healthy volunteers. The subsequent publication of his book, *DMT: The Spirit Molecule*, has enthused a whole new generation of interest in the subject of psychedelics.[30]

Franz X. Vollenweider is Director of Heffter Research Centre Zürich for Consciousness Studies (HRC-ZH). Vollenweider is also Vice-Director of Research and Teaching and Director of the Neuropsyhcopharmacology and Brain Imaging Research Unit of the University Hospital of Psychiatry Zürich East and Professor of Psychiatry in the School of Medicine. His contribution to the pre-clinical understanding of psychedelic drugs in recent years is invaluable, and he has published voluminously on their neurophysiology. He also gives marvellous lectures about neurotransmitters wherever he goes.

Anna Waldstein is a medical anthropologist who studies self-medication with herbal medicines as a form of empowerment and/or resistance to bio-medical hegemony. Her research interests include self-medication with cannabis and the relationship between cannabis and identity. She is also interested in the role of psychotropic substances in human evolution and biocultural constructions of addiction. She works at the University of Kent, Canterbury, and as co-chair was a driving force of organisation, inspiration and spiritual awareness for the 2011 Breaking Convention conference in the UK.

Charlotte Walsh is a lecturer at Leicester University, UK, where she teaches law and criminology. She has produced important work highlighting the legal aspects of the war on drugs, particularly pertaining to psychedelics and the issues of civil liberty and religious freedom.

Together with the reams of important people left off this list, these people are all continuing to contribute to the development of psychedelic research as a valid topic for mainstream scientific and social study in the twenty-first century and beyond. One thing all these people have in common is their ability to move seamlessly through the obscure world of today's psychedelic community while also being able to orientate themselves towards the more conservative environment of modern research platforms. The capacity to do this is essential if we are to see these compounds returning to mainstream practice and study.

CHAPTER 9

The Psychedelic Renaissance Part Two: Contemporary Studies

What do we want?
Evidence-based practice!
When do we want it?
After peer review!
— Banner held by anonymous protester at a 2011 Occupy March

When Did the Psychedelic Renaissance Begin?

The truth is psychedelic research never stopped entirely, but it certainly drastically reduced in volume and ceased being mainstream around about 1966 when LSD was made illegal. After this point, it was difficult to obtain a license to research or work clinically with psychedelic drugs. Sandoz also stopped distributing its product and recalled all remaining stocks from people who had stockpiled LSD, although, by then, many other places were synthesizing the drug (Czechoslovakia had a particularly good record for LSD manufacture). While these restrictions significantly reduced psychedelic research, not everyone gave up. There were a number of academic studies that continued for a while after the ban and Czech LSD research certainly continued at a sanatorium in Sadska until at least 1974.[1]

In the UK, any psychiatrists who still had supplies of LSD could continue prescribing it if they wished; and this carried on into the 1970s, with the last recorded dose being given to a patient in private practice in 1976. As noted, the next time a classical psychedelic was legally given to anyone in the UK was 33 years later when David Nutt injected me with psilocybin.

MDMA emerged in the late seventies and was used legally by a small handful of therapists right up to 1985. When it was banned, there followed a further 25 years of persistent campaigning to get the next MDMA human clinical research published.

So, of one sort or another. psychedelic research never completely went away. But what has happened in the last 20 years has been an unprecedented growth of psychedelic interest *within the mainstream*, which is what this renaissance is all about.

How to Get a Drug to Market

For those not familiar with how a research team gets a drug approved as a clinical medicine, I will give a very brief description of the process.[2]

Many clinical treatments in medicine first arise out of accidental anecdotal experience. Many others arise because a pharmaceutical company has specifically designed a new chemical with a particular target in mind. When a new chemical emerges in this way, there are pre-clinical studies that must be carried out in order to test whether the chemical is safe to be given to humans. *In vitro* tests involve adding concentrations of the chemical to isolated slices of tissues (heart, lungs, kidneys, brain, etc.) to determine the drug's toxicity. The new chemical will also be tested against animal models, which provides further information about safety and toxicity. This process of animal testing is highly controversial for many people outside the field of pharmacology and often arouses a strong emotional response.

The next part of the process is known as 'phase one clinical studies' in which the drug is tested on healthy human volunteers, that is, people without the specific disorder the drug is intended to treat. The purpose of such tests are to gather information about appropriate safe doses and subjective effects of the new drug. Volunteers, often students at the university where the research is being carried out, are usually paid for their services. I have taken part in lots of such trials, though never paid, because I find them interesting. Once this part is over, one can begin the phase two studies These involve small-scale clinical trials in which the drug is given to handfuls of patients with the disorder one is testing. Between 10 to 40 people is usual.

Clinical studies must be rigorously designed to reduce as many aspects of bias as possible. The gold standard for drug development is the double-blind placebo controlled randomised study in which identically matched subjects are randomly assigned into a control group or an experimental group. Then one group gets the active drug and the other gets the placebo drug (they look identical). Neither the subjects nor the examiners who will be testing the subjects' outcomes know which group has been given which drug. In this way, one hopes to claim that any differences seen in outcomes between the two groups can be put down entirely to the physiological action of the drug and not due to other influences.

After phase two comes phase three, in which the established best treatment regime with the new drug is rolled out to larger, multicentre groups for wide-scale testing on clinical patients. In this way, many hundreds of patients will receive treatment under a standardised protocol to ensure uniform results. From here the drug may then go out to market but under a very restricted license. Thousands of patients will get to use it in an open label fashion (that is, they know what they are taking, rather than blindly) and their doctors will closely monitor their process and document any adverse effects to the drug company.

The timescale and costs of the process described above are extremely variable. It can take between five and twenty years to get a drug to market in this way. Today the average cost of getting a brand new drug to market is around £75 million.

How This Research Method Relates to Psychedelic Drugs

The interesting thing about the psychedelic drugs is that we have literally tens of millions of cases of anecdotal uses of the drugs LSD, psilocybin, MDMA, ketamine, ibogaine, ayahuasca, cannabis and others over many decades — largely with safe and positive clinical effects. This is great, but because these 'clinical' uses have been occurring outside of the official clinical environment such cases are not enough for the regulatory authorities to immediately support these drugs becoming licensed medicines. And although people have been consuming these drugs for millennia and their toxicity profiles are low, we still have to carry out all the pre-clinical studies. Only once the drugs are deemed safe for human consumption can the phase one dosage studies on healthy volunteers take place. Then, if they are successful, the drug can go to phase two and then phase three studies.

One might have thought that the costs and timescales for getting psychedelic drugs to market ought to be quicker than for a newly invented chemical with no documented human use, but this is not the case. Although we already know the anecdotal use is relatively safe, this does not count as data sufficient for regulatory authorities. Furthermore, because the psychedelic drugs are all controlled or illegal drugs, one must have government approval to work with them, which means jumping through many legal and political loopholes and even putting up with unwanted media intrusions into one's research. The sum total of these unbelievably harsh regulatory processes applied to this kind of research makes the process prohibitively lengthy and costly — as we have seen earlier with the hard road from MDMA being banned in 1985 to the publication of the first phase two study in 2010.

It will be another good ten years before phase three trials are over for MDMA. In other words, MDMA, a drug which is not new, but rather one with a very well-known toxicity and record of safety at dosages recommended for therapy, will have taken at least 35 years to get to market, assuming it does make it by 2022.

Looking at the Contemporary Research for the Drugs

Below, we will look at each of the major psychedelic compounds in turn, outlining some of the published studies and discussing some of the future planned projects. It is a great pleasure to state that because of the rapidly expanding growth of this subject this section will be outdated even before it is published.

1. MDMA

Contemporary Clinical Research Completed
The majority of contemporary research with MDMA has centred on its role as an adjunct to trauma-focused psychotherapy for PTSD. I have described above in preceding chapters why MDMA is so perfectly suited for this kind of work. It is

almost as if the drug were designed with this purpose in mind (though this is not actually the case). Having experienced firsthand the massive difficulties in helping stuck patients with repressed and intrusive memories of severe psychological trauma, my colleagues and I are absolutely committed to putting ourselves behind this research.

To date there is only one clinical MDMA study completed and published, which is the PTSD study below by Michael Mithoefer et al, titled:

> The safety and efficacy of 3,4-methylenedioxymethamphetamine-assisted psychotherapy in subjects with chronic, treatment-resistant posttraumatic stress disorder: the first randomized controlled pilot study.[3]

Mithoefer and colleagues used MDMA-assisted psychotherapy on 20 patients with chronic PTSD, refractory to both psychotherapy and psychopharmacology. 12 patients received inactive placebo and eight received two or three sessions of MDMA (initial dose of 125mg followed after two hours by a further booster of 62.5mg). Both groups received a course of preparatory and follow-up non-drug psychotherapy. Using the Clinician-Administered PTSD Scale (CAPS) as a primary outcome measure, Mithoefer demonstrated that at two and twelve month follow-up 83% of the experimental group no longer met the criteria for PTSD, compared to just 25% of the patients in the placebo group. He also looked at neurocognitive and neurophysiological measures and showed that there were no drug-related serious adverse events, adverse neurocognitive effects or clinically significant blood pressure increases.

The Mithoefers' study has set a high benchmark for others to follow. Since the publication of this initial study in 2010, Michael has submitted the long-term follow-up, which is due for publication soon. It demonstrates that, even after up to four years since that single course of MDMA therapy, all the responders have continued to maintain the same rates of remission from PTSD.

Critic responses to their study — of which there have been many given the unbelievably good results they have shown — have ranged from comments about the impossibility of maintaining the blind control to the fact that the experimenters, by temperament, are so inspirational and positive that this has positively swayed the results, making them un-reproducible. Personally, I think their study, which is very well designed (especially as it is the first of it's kind in modern times), has illuminated a genuine positive clinical effect. But time will tell whether these results can be reproduced. And, as for Michael and Annie Mithoefer being inspirational people — there is not much that anyone can do about that except celebrate it and encourage them to train others in their methods — which is exactly what they are doing.

The MDMA/PTSD Switzerland Study by Oehen et al

Peter Oehen and Verena Widmer have been the co-therapists on this study, which has sought to reproduce the results seen by Mithoefer's study in the States. At the time of writing, the study is now complete, written up and the final paper has been submitted to the *Journal of Psychopharmacology* for consideration for publication

(I know this because I have been one of the reviewers). The results are certainly in favour of MDMA-assisted psychotherapy being more effective than placebo at reducing rates of PTSD, though not quite as spectacularly positive as those seen in the original Mithoefer study.

Aside from the single published Mithoefer study and the finished but unpublished Oehen study, there are a number of other MDMA clinical studies, two of which are described below, that didn't quite get off the ground. They are all available to view at the MAPS website.[4]

MDMA/PTSD Study in Spain

José Carlos Bouso in Madrid, Spain was running this study. It started in 1999, then, in 2002, after treating just six of 29 planned patients, the permission was revoked and the study was shut down because of political pressure. This stands as an illustration of the difficulties involved in carrying out psychedelic research in today's climate.

MDMA and Anxiety Secondary to Advanced Stage Cancer

This study by John Halpern at Harvard University began recruiting soon after it's approval in 2004. It was planned that twelve subjects with end-stage cancer and associated anxiety would undergo treatment with MDMA-assisted psychotherapy. But only one subject completed the study and after the second subject dropped out the study was closed due to enrolment challenges.

It is also worthy of note that Dr. Charles Grob's study of psilocybin therapy for end-stage cancer patients was originally planned for MDMA until it was felt that the regulatory barriers to using MDMA were considered insurmountable so Grob switched to psilocybin.

Future MDMA Studies Underway

The role of MDMA as an adjunct to psychotherapy for a range of mental health problems has now been opened-up by Mithoefer's study. Mithoefer's next project, already underway, is a study using MDMA-assisted psychotherapy specifically for veterans of war. This is a very important topic and a shrewd move on the part of Mithoefer and MAPS. The wars in Iraq and Afghanistan are taking their toll on the US and UK military personnel, nations at large, and, crucially, the politicians who are sending the troops to war. Governments are spending billions in disability payments for tens of thousands of sufferers of post-combat PTSD returning from warzones. It has become a medical, financial and political problem of growing proportions. The military is desperate for a way out, but the current treatments for PTSD are less than perfect and too many veterans are going untreated.

Some commentators have said there ought be no part for psychedelic research in helping out the military by adapting their methods specifically to treat veterans of war. But, thankfully, Doblin and Mithoefer — neither of them likely to be supporters of the wars themselves — do not see things this way. Rather, they accept that if the military is going to continue to do what it is doing, then someone has to be there to pick up the causalities. And if MDMA can offer a ray of hope to such hapless sufferers then that is all well and good.

If Mithoefer's latest project, aimed specifically at war veterans in the USA, is successful, it could open to the door to a very large population of desperate patients in need of effective treatment for PTSD.

MDMA/PTSD U.S. Relapse Study

Michael Mithoefer is also carrying out a study on those subjects from his original cohort that relapsed following their initial treatment with MDMA. The idea is to show that with some extra booster sessions the positive effects of the treatment can be maintained, even for those people that relapsed. It marks an important precedent because it demonstrates that we need not think of such treatments as having to be one-off magic bullets. After all, the current traditional treatments for PTSD involve taking *daily* SSRI drugs and carrying out multiple courses of trauma-focused psychotherapy. Why should it be, therefore, that MDMA-therapy only need happen once to be considered a success or a failure? This study by Mithoefer may set the trend for repeated courses of MDMA-assisted therapy for those subjects whose severity of PTSD warrants such an approach.

MDMA/PTSD U.S. Intern Study

This study being conducted by Marcela Otalora with support from MAPS is specifically aimed at training-up relatively inexperienced MDMA-psychotherapists in order that they can carry out MDMA-assisted therapy. This is an important new development and one that my colleagues and I have been keen to explore in the design of our UK-based MDMA project (see later). One criticism that could be aimed at Michael and Annie Mithoefer's study is that, between them, they are such an influential co-therapist pair of highly trained and experienced professionals that they are bound to yield great results — both for their experimental and placebo groups. However, if this kind of therapy is ever going to make it into mainstream medicine it is going to have to be reproducible by people with far less experience than the Mithoefers. Hence, this current study that looks to see how effectively interns can be trained-up to deliver this extremely idiosyncratic form of therapy.

International MDMA Research in the Pipeline

MAPS, Heffter and The Beckley Foundation are truly international. They are working with clinical teams all over the world to try to gather more data to back up the original Mithoefer Phase-Two study. The eventual plan is to move into phase-three studies within the next few years, with an eventual goal to see this form of PTSD treatment enter mainstream practice within the next 10 to 15 years. A number of international teams are attempting to recreate Michael's excellent results.

- In Australia a team lead by Stuart Saker and Fiona MacKenzie from Sydney are currently at the stage of working with MAPS to develop a protocol for their MDMA/PTSD study.

- In Canada Ingrid Pacey and Andrew Feldmar from Vancouver have had their study approved and are awaiting their permit to import the MDMA so their study can begin.
- In Israel MAPS is working with a clinical team awaiting FDA approval before further planning of their MDMA/PTSD Phase Two study.
- In Jordan a team lead by Nasser Shuriquie from Amman is awaiting Jordanian approval to begin their study.

The UK MDMA/PTSD Study: Its Development and Growth

For at least five years, since meeting Michael Mithoefer at the ENCP conference in Vienna, I have been talking to MAPS about a wish to develop a UK-based phase-two MDMA-assisted psychotherapy for PTSD study. We have been through a number of different ideas before settling on our current approach. A big problem at first was finding a group of psychotherapists and psychologists willing to work on such a project. I never had any problems gathering the psychopharmacology support (having had David Nutt on board from the beginning), but the psychotherapy side was proving more challenging.

Then I met Jonathan Bisson in 2009 when I was invited with Mithoefer and Grob to convene a panel on psychedelic therapy for the Royal College of Psychiatrists annual conference in Liverpool. Bisson is the lead of a large clinical research facility at Cardiff University, which specialises on cases of post-trauma. He sees hundreds of new cases every year with PTSD, many secondary to post-combat trauma.

I met with Bisson and discussed my plans for an MDMA study. Bisson, who is ex-services himself, is an open-minded doctor with a passionate interest to try anything that could reliably work to improve the treatment rates for PTSD. With David Nutt also involved to provide psychopharmacology support and add an element of neuroimaging to the study, everything was in place.

Although, in principle, the purpose of our study is to add to the raft of phase-two studies following in the wake of Mithoefer's, ours differs in as much as we are keen to demonstrate that with just minimal training any standard NHS clinic anywhere could deliver this treatment. We feel this is an essential component if we are to convince the regulatory authorities that it is not only experienced and inspirational experts like Mithoefer and Oehen that can make this therapy work.

At the time of writing we are finalising the outline protocol and waiting for funding. I hope by the time this book is published the study will be underway.

Original Ideas for New MDMA Research

So far, I have restricted all talk about MDMA therapy to its use as an agent to manage PTSD, but that need not be the limit of its effectiveness as a clinical agent. Indeed, there are some other theoretical uses for MDMA described below. No such projects are even underway yet but watch this space, as in the next ten years I am sure they will be.

MDMA for Depression

What about MDMA for depression? MDMA has a very clear effect on raising mood and improving feelings of wellbeing. After all, that is why 300,000 kids every weekend in the UK take the drug recreationally. But what happens when depressed people take MDMA?[5] Because of the gap in our knowledge about therapeutic applications for MDMA, this question cannot yet be answered with confidence. The theoretical potential of using MDMA as a potent serotonin-enhancer to treat depression has been postulated by Riedlinger and Montagne in a chapter in Julie Holland's *Ecstasy* book.[6] But there is very little empirical clinical information regarding the effects of MDMA on depressed patients. There exist numerous anecdotal reports of the expected transient rise in mood during recreational use of MDMA by depressed people, but this is often followed by a subsequent depressed mood and other associated unpleasant psychological and physiological 'hangover' effects. Because of these negative effects, there is little evidence — anecdotal or otherwise — of depressed people carrying out long-term self-medication with MDMA.

The existence of a hangover associated with MDMA is well documented by recreational users of ecstasy. Among ecstasy users, this hangover effect (sometimes called the 'mid-week blues' or 'blue Wednesday'), may last for between one and seven days, but it is certainly exacerbated by the adverse environmental circumstances in which recreational ecstasy is often consumed (i.e., at night with consequent sleep deprivation, missing meals, excessive physical exertion and often being taken with other psychoactive drugs, including alcohol).

There is certainly a place for a trial that examines the possible role for MDMA in treating depression. Recreationally, and in the current MDMA-assisted psychotherapy studies, subjects tend to use doses of 120mg plus. But it is not known what effect the drug may have if taken at much smaller dosages (say 10–25mg) for longer periods of time. Taken repeatedly at these lower doses, could MDMA have a gradual, beneficial effect on mood? Perhaps a trial that proposed administering 'sub-psychedelic' doses of MDMA, on a regular basis, to patients with clinical depression might be of benefit. One might expect the drug to have similar effects to the SSRI drugs, but because one need not wait for serotonin levels to build up slowly through inhibiting re-uptake of the neurotransmitter, one might propose the mood-enhancing effects of low-dose MDMA might be noticed much quicker than with an SSRI drug. And perhaps, if taken in such low doses, there might not be such a dramatic rebound serotonin depletion causing a significant hangover effect. The possibility of using MDMA to lift mood early and then transfer to an SSRI of other antidepressant to continue longer term might be considered. Watch out to see if this sort of research emerges to explore whether MDMA could be developed as an antidepressant.

MDMA as an Alternative to ECT

One particular area where MDMA's rapid onset of action may be of use clinically is in circumstances where mood elevation is required quickly for emergency reasons and there is no time to wait for up to six weeks for the antidepressant effects of traditional drugs. In these situations, the current treatment is electro-convulsive therapy (ECT). In this scenario, could MDMA be used instead of ECT?[5]

ECT, like psychedelic therapy, is one of those great areas of psychiatry where there exist many erroneous preconceptions in the general public that have the net result of withholding an effective, safe, cheap and relatively unobtrusive treatment from those patients who might otherwise benefit from it. The general public's understanding of ECT is appallingly bad. This is the case, at least, in the Western world. It is of note that in many non-Western countries they queue up for ECT, which they do not consider to be nearly as barbaric as we do in the West (perhaps because the 1976 film *One Flew Over the Cuckoo's Nest* was not seen so prolifically). Indeed, in India the general public consider the practice of taking daily doses of drugs as treatments for depression — as we are so prone to do here — to be far more invasive and unsavoury than a few quick and effective doses of electricity. So the idea that ECT is a bad thing is not universally the case. This illustrates well that our opinions are often based not on any particular evidence, but on where we live and what sort of propaganda we have been exposed to. All though I am sure some people within the profession of psychiatry would disagree with me, the vast majority of those with experience of working with severe mental illness will generally opt to choose ECT for resistant depression, as evidenced by a survey in which the majority of Indian psychiatrists themselves said it would be their first choice if they had severe depression.[7]

In the West, we reserve ECT only for the most severe cases, those in which other treatments have failed or in which we need a rapid serotonin rush to kick-start someone out of the depths of severe — often catatonic — depression in which, by refusing food, the sufferer risks death by starvation. I have always been interested to know what would happen if you gave a high dose (say 150mg) of MDMA to a severely depressed catatonic patient. Who knows? My guess is that it would rapidly bounce them out of their catatonic state. If so, it could be life saving.

So this is another study to look out for in coming years. Furthermore, because ECT is generally seen as such an unsavoury thing in the West then I believe a study that could be billed as 'the nail in the coffin for ECT' might get easily approved and supported.

MDMA for Autism
The idea of using MDMA to treat autism is a reasonable proposition. Indeed, such a study is most likely not at all far away. In January 2012, MAPS put out an invite for researchers to come forward to study the role that MDMA could have as a treatment for autism and they offered $10,000 to a clinical team who wish to instigate such a study.[8]

Those with experience of autism — which certainly includes all child psychiatrists — will know that this is a spectrum of clinical disorders that share the common characteristics of restricted ranges of interest (obsessional behavioural or repetitive habits), impaired social functioning (characterised by a lack of understanding of social cues, rules and manners), impaired communication, and abnormal use of language. At the more severe end of the spectrum (sometimes called 'full blown autism'), sufferers may have learning difficulties and no development of speech and language at all. At the other end of the spectrum (sometimes called high-functioning autism or Asperger's Syndrome, although they are not quite the same thing), a person may have an abnormally high intelligence and very advanced language use but still suffer with social functioning difficulties and a tendency to be overly pedantic and inflexible. A fictional account of adult autism is given in the film *Rain Man*.

One of the cardinal features of autism is a tendency for a sufferer to lack empathy. That is, they do not appear to recognise the emotional responses of others and may appear aloof and disinterested in other people's worlds. In this book, we have already described how MDMA has a particular effect to increase levels of empathy in the user.

MAPS' call to get such a study started comes out of the observed anecdotal effect that autistic adults who have used ecstasy recreationally appear to demonstrate reduced empathy impairments during, and for some time after, the intoxication with the drug. This is certainly an avenue worthy of further study. The current treatments for autism are largely either educational, social, functional or purely symptomatic — with the full range of psychiatric drugs used as and when they are needed. If MDMA can offer a way out of the 'locked in/locked out' aspect of social impairments secondary to autism, it would be greatly welcomed by those clinicians working with the condition.[9]

Could MDMA-psychotherapy be Applied to Borderline Personality Disorder?

Aside from PTSD, as it appears in it's 'simple' form (associated with discrete trauma such as post-combat-PTSD), a slight variation of the diagnosis is increasingly pervading psychiatry. It is now being applied in an expanded form as 'complex-PTSD', which refers to a history of trauma in which a person might not have had a single necessarily *life-threatening* traumatic episode, but might have suffered multiple episodes of non-life-threatening but equally frightening experiences of trauma — such as repetitive episodes of child sexual abuse. Such a history can lead to an emotionally unstable (for example, borderline) personality disorder (BPD), which is often very difficult to treat.

There are high rates of treatment resistance for BPD because the effects of repeated abuse render the sufferer highly prone to dissociative episodes in which they readily re-experience the frightening memories of their abuse. Whenever they attempt to 'go back there' in their thoughts, they dissociate, which may happen spontaneously at any time of the day or in their nightmares. This makes undergoing trauma-focused psychotherapy (where the subject is *expected* to reflect upon their experience of abuse) extremely difficult. In such cases, an agent such as MDMA could be useful.

Clinically, I have seen many teenage girls with emerging BPD. They so often present with a horrendous clinical picture of repetitive self-harm and suicide attempts. They have all the hallmark features of PTSD (hypervigilance, avoidance of cues that remind them of their abuse, flashbacks and nightmares), as well as drug and alcohol problems and a worrying tendency to seek out new abusive relationships that maintain them in the cycle of trauma. All of this develops as an attempt to mask the symptoms of PTSD. It is very difficult to treat these girls because they are so terrified of their memories of trauma that they go out of their way to avoid therapies aimed at encouraging them to discuss their past. Their sense of being stuck is painful to watch. and I have known several tragic cases of girls committing suicide despite all their own hard work and good intentions, as well as the help and support of their families, their social workers and the committed psychiatric staff caring for them.

In the current MDMA PTSD studies, there have always been careful exclusion criteria to avoid enrolling patients with too many rigid borderline tendencies. This is understandable, as the last thing researchers need at this crucial early stage of modern psychedelic research is patients suffering episodes of high-profile self-harm or even completed suicide. Mithoefer and others have intentionally shied away from such risky patients and excluded them when writing their protocols, and who can blame them?

Ultimately, however, this is the group of patients I would like to help the most with MDMA-assisted psychotherapy. I think it could be just what is needed to allow these fragile and desperate people the kind of psychological protection they need to allow them to break through their heavily fortified defences; it might enable them to stare their histories of abuse in the face, while feeling sufficiently bolstered by MDMA's effects to be able to do the trauma-focused work.

MDMA has unique properties to augment trauma-focused psychotherapy. It acts like a life raft or a rubber ring. It can buffer the most intense and frightening aspects of the traumatic memories, yet it still allows the patient to experience enough of the pain to carry out real-time trauma-focused psychotherapy. This is a hugely valuable tool for patients who, up until now, have been unable to approach their past without being overwhelmed by negative affect and subsequently fleeing the therapy, back into their 'safe' world of self-harm, drug abuse and severe self-neglect.

This does not mean that trauma-focused therapy with MDMA is a walk in the park. Indeed, one of Mithoefer's patients told him, 'I don't know why they call this ecstasy!' Under MDMA-therapy, these traumatised patients certainly do still experience the pain of their memories. But the MDMA acts as cushion to make doing this work possible. And as a psychiatrist who has seen too many young patients give up their fight against their past, I am very excited by the prospect of a clinical tool that can do this.

2. LSD

This next section on completed clinical studies with LSD is short. As it stands, at the time of writing there are *no* contemporary published clinical studies with LSD psychotherapy and only a couple of review papers discussing the role for LSD as an analgesic agent. This is despite an extensive history of LSD psychotherapy and many thousands of papers written during the 1950s and 60s describing it's use — from Sandison, Grof, Leary, Osmond, Hoffer, Fadiman, Stolaroff and countless others.

There are several reasons why LSD has not been studied more extensively during the latest psychedelic renaissance, some of which are psychopharmacological but mostly of which are political. Many contemporary studies in which the researchers wanted to use a 'classical' psychedelic have opted for psilocybin rather than LSD. This may be because psilocybin is slightly easier to use than LSD; it is shorter acting, less cumbersome for a clinical study involving many patients and repeated sessions with the drug, and the high itself is generally a little less intense and perceptually distorting (though many would challenge this). But the main reason why researchers have opted for psilocybin is simply that LSD has such a widely known reputation as a negative drug in the eyes of the media, politicians, ethics boards and parents everywhere, which has a detrimental effect on obtaining a research license and funding. Many lay people, while perhaps familiar with magic mushrooms, have not heard of the drug psilocybin, which makes it an altogether easier proposition to use for a study in which researchers are keen to avoid unwanted media intrusions.

Basically, then, some 40 years since the dreaded 'psychedelic sixties' came to an end, those three little letters L.S.D. are still enough to strike fear into people's hearts and make research very difficult indeed.

Peter Gasser's LSD Study

Because of the reasons described above — and in homage to Albert Hofmann — when the Swiss psychotherapist Peter Gasser designed his clinical trial of psychedelic-drug assisted psychotherapy for the treatment of anxiety associated with end-stage cancer, he was determined to not give in and choose psilocybin. He insisted on using LSD. Gasser was keen to get his study off the ground during Hoffman's lifetime, which he achieved. Hofmann died in 2008 after a lifetime dedicated to psychedelic research in which he saw his creation, LSD, initially hailed as a 'wonder drug' in the 1950s, turn into a 'problem child' in the 1960s and then almost entirely disappear from view in modern medicine.

Gasser was granted permission to carry out his study in December 2007, prompting Hofmann to say: 'My wish has come true. I didn't think I'd live to find out that LSD had finally taken its place in medicine'.

The Gasser study, which is sponsored by MAPS, has finished collecting data and is currently at the stage of being written-up and submitted for publication. Gasser uses high doses (200 mcg) of LSD in a double-blind method for 12 patients with end-stage cancer. The LSD experience lends itself perfectly to the kind of existential experiences that go with a person coming to terms with their death from cancer.[10] The scientific world eagerly awaits the publication of this work.

LSD as an Analgesic for Treating Cluster Headaches

It has long been known anecdotally that the classical psychedelic drugs LSD and psilocybin, when used recreationally, have a positive analgesic effect at treating the severe pain associated with cluster headaches. This incredibly disabling condition has sometimes been referred to as 'suicide headaches' because the intensity of pain has been known to drive some sufferers to kill themselves.

Yet frequently, when people take small, sub-psychedelic doses of LSD or magic mushrooms, not only does their headache disappear during the course of the intoxication, but also for many weeks or even months afterwards. The mechanism for how this works is not fully understood but it probably relates to the classical psychedelics role as central vasoregulators. The anaesthetist Eric Kast discovered these analgesic effects of LSD in the 1960s. He carried out studies with the drug and found it to be more effective and better tolerated than traditional opiate-based analgesics.[11]

In modern times, the idea to study cluster headache sufferers arose when, in 2004 the internet-based support group Clusterbusters approached MAPS and asked them to evaluate the large numbers of anecdotal reports that the website was getting about the usefulness of recreational classical psychedelics for relieving cluster headache pain. A subsequent review of these cases by Andrew Sewell, John Halpern and Harrison Pope has now lead to a new study being planned, to be led by Halpern at Harvard and sponsored by MAPS.[12] Together with Torsten Passie at Medizinische Hoschule Hannover in Germany, John Halpern has also been in the process of developing a non-psychedelic analogue (2-Bromo-LSD, or 'BOL') to be used as an alternative to the hallucinogenic effects of LSD. The results of their recent pilot study with BOL were published as a poster abstract at the 2011 International Headache Conference.[13]

The implications for this work could be far-reaching and stretch well beyond psychiatry. Because it seems that the drugs exert their analgesic effects at such low doses and without the need for specialised psychedelic psychotherapy, this kind of psychopharmacology research could radically rewrite the textbooks as far as standard analgesia for general medicine goes.

3. Psilocybin

In recent years, psilocybin has risen to the top of the list as the classical psychedelic substance with greatest potential for clinical research for the reasons mentioned above. There have been a number of important studies looking specifically at the role for the drug in treating anxiety disorders and some highly significant non-clinical studies have pushed forward our understanding of essential neurophysiological processes and the nature of consciousness. And it looks like there is much more to come.

Psilocybin to Treat Obsessive Compulsive Disorder

It has long been known anecdotally that many sufferers with obsessive-compulsive disorder (OCD) frequently show a spontaneous remission of symptoms, sometimes lasting several weeks, when they take LSD or magic mushrooms. When MAPS sponsored this double-blind placebo-controlled pilot study by Francisco Moreno at the University of Arizona in 2006, it became the first piece of clinical psilocybin research since 1970.[14] Moreno looked at nine patients with severe OCD, which had not responded to traditional treatments. Psilocybin was shown to substantially reduce OCD symptoms in several of the patients, one for several weeks after the treatment.

It is just early days in the research of this approach to OCD with psilocybin, but there is certainly more to come in this field in the future. Unremitting OCD is a very disabling and difficult to treat condition. Patients — and their psychiatrists — will welcome any new and innovative approach that is likely to contribute to the management of the disorder.

Psilocybin to Treat Anxiety Associated with End-stage Cancer[15]

This study by Charles Grob, Professor of Child and Adolescent Psychiatry at the Harbor-UCLA Medical Center, Torrance, California, started out with the proposal to use MDMA as the active agent, but Grob then switched to psilocybin because the apparently insurmountable regulatory problems associated at that time with MDMA research.

There is a rich history of using psychedelics to assist patients with the existential issues associated with dying, with much of the work in this field being done by Stanislav Grof and Joan Halifax in the 1960s. Charlie Grob's study became the first psychedelic treatment with terminally ill patients since the early 1970s. All of the patients in the study had end-stage cancer and were experiencing unremitting anxiety. Using a double-blind placebo-controlled method, Grob demonstrated that psilocybin-assisted psychotherapy reduced psycho-spiritual anxiety, depression, and physical pain for these patients.

Of note, another psilocybin clinical study for sufferers of cancer is currently underway by Roland Griffiths' team at Johns Hopkins University. In this study 44 patients will be treated with psilocybin-assisted psychotherapy. It is similar to Grob's study, but Griffiths will be working with early-stage as well as late-stage cancer patients. Similar outcome measures will be employed as Griffiths is hoping to show that psilocybin relieves the pain associated with cancer as well as improving quality of life and helping patients to overcome the anxiety and existential crises associated with their diagnosis of cancer.

Important Non-clinical Contemporary Psilocybin Research

There are lots of pre-clinical and neurophysiological studies conducted in recent years, many of which have come out of the laboratories of Franz Vollenweider and Dave Nichols from projects overseen by the Heffter Research Institute on both sides of the Atlantic. Below are described two important non-clinical studies that are having profound effects on the way we view consciousness and spirituality. They will also have an important impact on the future of clinical research.

Psilocybin: The Spiritual Experience and Personality Change

I have already alluded to this piece of work throughout this book. It was carried out by Roland Griffiths, Bill Richards et al at Johns Hopkins School of Medicine and published in 2006.[16] Some call it a recreation or re-visitation of the famous Good Friday Experiment by Walter Pahnke, but there were some significant differences.

Griffiths took a group of 30 healthy volunteers who had never before taken a psychedelic drug before and gave them alternate sessions with either high-dose psilocybin (30mg orally) or an identical-looking placebo capsule of methylpheni-date, which provided a light stimulating effect to fool the user into thinking they had taken an active drug, but with no psychedelic effect. Sessions were spaced two-months apart and rating scales were used to test subjects' appreciation of drug effects and mystical experience at three stages: immediately after each session, at two months after the session and at fourteen months follow-up. It was a double-blind study, with neither subjects nor examiners knowing whether each person had received the psilocybin or the placebo during each session. Sessions, which lasted an average of eight hours each, were carried out individually in a relaxed and sup-portive environment with minimal interventions from the investigators. Mainly, subjects usually chose to lie down and relax with eye-shades on, listening to music. They were encouraged to simply just 'go inside their heads'.

The results showed that 61% of the psilocybin group versus 13% of the control group reported a 'complete mystical experience'. Notably, one third of subjects also described the psilocybin experience as unpleasant and anxiety provoking at times. All the subjects taking high-dose psilocybin considered it a deeply profound experience, with one third describing it as 'the single most spiritually significant event of their lives' and two thirds saying it was 'among their five most meaningful and spiritually significant events'. These results were sustained: at 14 months after the last session, the psilocybin group continued to attribute deep personal meaning to the experience. Roland Griffiths has gone on to publish further results as a spin-off from this initial study. More recent papers have described how the optimum dose for a mystical or spiritual experience is between 20mg and 30mg of psilocy-bin. Any less than this does not produce such a profound effect but higher doses than this are overly anxiety-provoking.

But perhaps the most interesting results to come out of this work by Griffiths and Richards are those that relate to the subtle but lasting personality changes that have occurred in the cohort of subjects who experienced high-dose psilocybin for the first time in his study. The investigators measured the long-term effects of the treatment on five broad domains of personality: neuroticism, extroversion, open-ness, agreeableness, and conscientiousness. Subjects frequently reported increases in their aesthetic appreciation, imagination, and creativity and there were lasting observable increases in the domain of openness following a high-dose psilocybin session.[17]

The potential importance of these results is profound. It is the first time that sci-ence has demonstrated a phenomenon that is anecdotally obvious, namely, that a spiritually significant mystical experience predicts changes in behaviours, atti-tudes and values that are positive and long-lasting. The reason this has such great importance in psychiatry — and of particular interest to me — is that it relates to my earlier comments about those patients with personality disorder who had no apparent hope of a way out of their condition. An old adage in psychiatry, but one that is increasingly being challenged, is that 'once your (maladaptive or func-tional) personality has been formed nothing can change it'. Such a negative and fatalistic statement grates with every psychiatrist who has seen patients suffering because their ingrained personality appears to resist to any attempts to relieve them of their suffering. If psilocybin can seriously lead to long-lasting positive personality change — which many would claim is certainly the case anecdotally — this is an avenue worthy of much more exploration.

And finally, regarding Griffith's work, another important addition to his recent psilocybin research is the study he is now planning using psilocybin-assisted psychotherapy to combat nicotine addiction. If that study turns out to have positive results, the implications for helping smokers quit their addictions could be great. Cigarette addiction is thought to be the most prolific and difficult to treat (harder to break than heroin) and in the UK some 600,000 deaths occur every years from nicotine use. It really does require nothing short of a shift in one's personality to break the habit. Does the answer lie in a drug like psilocybin?'

Psilocybin and the Beyond Within

Two recent studies by Robin Carhart-Harris and colleagues at Imperial University using functional Magnetic Resonance Imaging (fMRI) have looked at psilocybin on healthy volunteers. While working with Carhart-Harris in Bristol, I was privileged to have helped out with and co-authored the dose-tolerability pilot study that preceded the actual imaging studies. In the pilot, we tested volunteers on different does of intravenous psilocybin while they lay inside a wooden mock MRI scanner. I regret being unable to be more involved in the following imaging study, other than volunteering as a healthy subject for the sessions that took place in Cardiff. But I did eventually get to review and approve the second paper for publication in *The Journal of Psychopharmacology*.

The basic rationale for Carhart-Harris' first fMRI psilocybin project was to measure the functional activity in the medial prefrontal cortex after psilocybin.[18] Large decreases in activity and blood flow were observed, contrary to popular assumptions that under the influence of psychedelic drugs there is an increase in brain blood flow and activity. Because the medial prefrontal cortex is known to exert a top-down inhibitory control over limbic activity (the site of the brain that governs emotional experiences), it was postulated that a psilocybin-induced deactivation of the medial prefrontal cortex leads to a disinhibition of limbic activity and an associated increased emotional response.

In the second study using fMRI, the investigators measured the subjective psychological effects of psilocybin when a subject was experiencing recall of positive emotional memories.[19] Ten healthy participants received two functional magnetic resonance imaging scans (2mg intravenous psilocybin versus intravenous saline), separated by approximately seven days, during which they viewed two different sets of positive autobiographical memory cues. Participants viewed each cue for 6 seconds ('early phase') and then closed their eyes for 16 seconds and imagined re-experiencing the event ('late phase'). In both conditions (psilocybin and placebo), statistically significant neural activations to the memories were seen in limbic and striatal regions in the early phase and the medial prefrontal cortex in the late phase. However, there were additional visual and other sensory cortical activations in the late phase under psilocybin that were absent under placebo. Subjects also gave ratings of the memory vividness and visual imagery that was significantly higher after psilocybin compared to placebo. An interpretation of these results is that psilocybin enhances autobiographical recollection — and this can be demonstrated objectively by observed brain functioning changes, which correlate with the subjectively reported psychological experience of increased recall and vividness.

The reason this result is so important for psychiatry is that it finally proves what has been known anecdotally for the last 60 years, since psychotherapists first began using LSD as a tool to enhance psychotherapy, namely, that *psychedelic drugs increase access to repressed emotional memories.* This is extremely helpful for any future psychotherapy studies being studied. Carhart-Harris has demonstrated graphically that this is how these drugs work.

The Future for Psilocybin Research

Another important finding that came out of Carhart-Harris' fMRI research was that psilocybin reduced neural activity in a part of the brain that has been shown in the past to be particularly over-active in depressed patients. This points the way to a study exploring whether there may be a role for the drug as an antidepressant. Robin Carhart-Harris and David Nutt at Imperial University are currently seeking funding for such a study. They are also exploring what effects psilocybin has on electrical brain activity, measuring magnetoencephalography (MEG) responses to healthy subjects under the influence of intravenous psilocybin. And I must confess this latest project of Carhart-Harris' has given me yet another excuse recently to make that trek to Cardiff and enjoy a particularly colourful train journey home.

4. Dimethyltryptamine (DMT)

Since Rick Strassman's pioneering human DMT study of 1995 launched the new renaissance of psychedelic research, there have been very few other published human studies of its use.[20] One paper, however, by Daumann et al in 2008, describes a study in which healthy human volunteers were given both DMT and ketamine under fMRI conditions.[21] This paper explores the potential role for DMT as a psychotomimetic to assist researchers developing psychopharmacological models for studying schizophrenia. (Funny how things come back into fashion isn't it?) The study suggests ketamine makes for a better psychotomimetic than DMT because the former mimics both positive and negative symptoms of schizophrenia whereas the latter only models the positive symptoms.

Another important recent pre-clinical DMT study is by Fontanilla et al, published in the journal *Science* in 2009, which postulated that DMT binds to the sigma-1 receptor in the brain.[22] This is an important discovery because the sigma-1 receptor was previously considered an 'orphan receptor', as no endogenous chemical had been found that binds to it. In their biochemical, physiological, and behavioural experiments with mice, they suggest DMT is an endogenous agonist for the sigma-1 receptor. This opens up the debate further made by McKenna, Strassman and others about endogenous DMT.

5. Ayahuasca

While human studies with pure DMT have been few and far between since Strassman's study, a lot of contemporary research with DMT in the form of ayahuasca is taking place. Numerous scholars have been at looking at the anthropological and social aspects of ayahuasca in non-Western cultures, how this relates to the stability of those populations and how it is increasingly emerging as a tool for self-exploration and healing in the West. For an excellent extensive review of many of the older and more contemporary studies with ayahuasca, see Dennis McKenna's review of research and developments.[23]

Another newer study worth mentioning here includes that by Joel Porfírio Pinto of the University of Sao Paulo, who, in 2010, published his thesis studying the fMRI, SPECT scans and neuropsychological changes in healthy volunteers given ayahuasca. SPECT showed activation of the frontal and temporal cortex and limbic areas. Cerebral blood flow decreased in a region of the right cerebellar hemisphere, and fMRI data showed decreased activation of areas involved in language processing. Pinto suggests ayahuasca could be useful for the study of the neurobiology of psychosis.[24] There are further series of pre-clinical and neurophysiological studies with ayahuasca that have been carried out by Jordi Riba in Spain. Details are given on the MAPS website.

In 2005 Charles Grob and Marlene Dobkin de Rios published a qualitative evaluation of Brazilian teenagers of the União do Vegetal Church who ritually use ayahuasca and compared them to local matched non-users. Data showed that the ayahuasca-using teenagers appeared to be healthy, thoughtful, considerate and bonded to their families and religious peers, with no evidence of any harm caused by their use of the plant compounds.[25]

Also in South America, there is currently a long-term evaluation being sponsored by MAPS of the very well established ayahuasca treatment program at the Takiwasi Center in Peru. The director of Takiwasi, Jacques Mabit, also wrote a good review of the history and on-going efforts at the centre in the 2007 book *Hallucinogens and* Health.[26]

And for even more reading on the anthropological aspects of human development alongside ayahuasca it is always a pleasure to read Graham Hancock's book *Supernatural: Meetings with the Ancient Teachers of Mankind.*[27]

6. Ketamine

Ketamine to Combat Addictions

The burden of alcohol abuse in Britain in horrendous, with 8,000 deaths each year, one person in twelve dependent on alcohol, 20% of suicides and 65% of suicide attempts related to alcoholism, up to 1.3 million children adversely affected by family drinking, around 35% of accident and emergency attendance and ambulance costs alcohol related and drink driving responsible for 17% of all road deaths.[28]

The current treatments for alcohol dependence are not great. A meta-analysis conducted ten years ago looked at 361 controlled studies and ranked treatment modalities. Top of the list was the 'brief intervention approach', followed by 'motivational enhancement' and two different pharmacotherapies: GABA agonist treatment (e.g., acamprosate) and opiate antagonists (e.g., naltrexone). Those approaches that attempted to simply educate or shock fared the least effective at reducing rates of alcoholism.[29]

So how good are acamprosate and naltrexone for treating alcoholism? A meta-analysis of 20 controlled trials involving 4000 patients treated with acamprosate showed that at 12 months abstinence rates were 27% for acamprosate compared to 13% for placebo, so basically not that great.[30] And a meta-analysis of 24 trials for naltrexone treatment only found significantly improved abstinence rates for the first 12 weeks and no differences between placebo and naltrexone at 12 months.[31] When acamprosate and naltrexone are combined, results are slightly better, with up to 73% abstinence after 12-weeks treatment period compared to just 20% on placebo. But this rate of improvement had dropped to 66% at three-month follow-up and by 12 months combined treatment was no better than naltrexone alone.[32] In summary, medical treatments for alcohol dependency, after a hundred years of concerted efforts by specialists, like many other psychiatric treatments, remains relatively poor and is sorely in need of an innovative approach.

What About Ketamine?

So far the majority of contemporary psychiatric research with ketamine has focused on its capacity to treat addictions. In this regard, the work of Evgeny Krupitsky, the Clinical Director of Research for the Saint Petersburg Regional Center for Research in Addiction and Psychopharmacology, has set out the way. In the 1990s, he developed a model of ketamine-assisted psychotherapy to treat alcohol and opiate addictions.

Krupitsky and Grinenko compared 111 alcoholic patients treat with ketamine-assisted psychotherapy (KPT) with 100 alcoholic patients treat with conventional treatment.[33] 66% of those treat with ketamine-assisted psychotherapy (KPT) remained sober after one year, compared to 24% of the control group. Krupitsky, who I met at a conference in Vienna in 2007, then invited to speak at Breaking Convention 2011, puts a lot of faith in the induction of a spiritual experience to explain his good results, which fits with the importance of the mystical experience to effect positive personality change.

Krupitsky further developed his technique and applied it to treating heroin addiction. He showed that one single session of KPT (compared to a placebo session) was enough to significantly promote improved abstinence from heroin for one year without any adverse reactions. He went on to study whether follow-up sessions with two further monthly KPT sessions after discharge from hospital following this initial KPT session improved long-term outcomes compared to those randomly allocated into a placebo group. At one-year follow-up there was a significantly higher rate of in the multiple KPT group, with 50% of subjects remaining abstinent from heroin compared to just 22% in the single KPT group.[34]

Krupitsky, although the most prolific, is not the only researcher to study the use of ketamine as a tool to improve addiction treatment. Another extraordinary study by Jovaisa et al. from Lithuania used low-dose ketamine, without combining it with psychotherapy, to demonstrate how the effects of the drug reduce the unpleasant withdrawal symptoms of heroin addiction.[35]

Ketamine as a Psychotomimetic and as an Antidepressant

As mentioned earlier, ketamine has been studied in recent years as a potential psychotomimetic to improve our understanding of schizophrenia and assist in the development of new antipsychotics. To appreciate how this works, one must first understand that ketamine is an NMDA-antagonist (a glutamate receptor antagonist) and that it mimics both positive and negative symptoms of schizophrenia. This has led psychopharmacologists to search for an effective glutamate receptor *agonist* as a potential treatment for psychosis. Using this ketamine psychotomimetic hypothesis as a model in healthy human subjects, we can give ketamine, induce psychotic symptoms and then test potential antipsychotic drugs against these induced effects. The role that ketamine plays in this kind of research can significantly push forward our understanding of schizophrenia (just as LSD did in the 1950s). This was carried out for the first time successfully in a recent study by D'Souza et al.[36]

Several recent contemporary publications suggest there may be a role for ketamine in the future of antidepressant developments. The first is a simple case series involving just two patients who coincidentally showed reductions in pre-existing depressive symptoms when being given injections of ketamine for a different condition (Complex Regional Pain Syndrome).[37] In another study, which was randomised, double blind and placebo controlled, a single injection of ketamine significantly improved symptoms in depressed patients who had been taken off all their usual antidepressant medication for up to a week. The effect size was large and the ketamine treatment was well tolerated.[38] This study by Zarate opens up an interesting new line of research in treating depression. Most antidepressants up till now have concentrated on raising levels of the monoamines (particularly serotonin and noradrenaline), but ketamine, which exerts its effects by glutamate inhibition — perhaps via increased activity at AMPA receptors — is getting a lot of psychiatrists talking right now. The concept that depression could be managed by a monthly or fortnightly injection, rather than having to take daily antidepressant tablets, is revolutionary. It is not unlike dialysis for the brain.

7. Ibogaine

Returning to the psychedelics' capacity for treating addictions, the drug ibogaine has long been known to combat addiction to alcohol, as evidenced by much lower rates of alcoholism in native ibogaine-using cultures. Alper et al recently highlighted several pre-clinical animal studies describing its effectiveness as an agent to combat addiction.[39]

In an open-label (not placebo controlled) study by Alper, ibogaine was explored as a treatment for opiate dependence. 33 patients with previous intravenous heroin addiction were given a single dose of ibogaine on stopping their opiate drugs. 25 of them showed a resolution of the signs of opiate withdrawal within 24 hours, which was maintained for a total of 72 hours.[40]

In recent years, ibogaine treatment clinics, both underground and licensed, have sprung up all over the world. MAPS is currently sponsoring research at ibogaine clinics in Mexico (with investigator Thomas Brown) and in New Zealand (with investigator Geoff Noller). These observational studies are gathering data about outcomes of long-running clinical programs. There are also treatment programs underway in Canada being evaluated by Leah Martin and Sandra Karpetas and in the UK.[41]

And it is not only alcohol and opiates that are purported to benefit from ibogaine treatment; increasing reports about its efficacy at combating cocaine addiction and methamphetamine abuse are also emerging.[42]

Contemporary Underground Therapy with Multiple Psychedelics

In 2010 David Nutt put me in touch with a mature and experienced German psychotherapist who had recently been released from prison. Friederike Fischer was trained as a psycholytic therapist during the legal loophole period of 1988 to 1993 in Switzerland. But when the group folded she was not content to let all that hard work go to waste, so she took the brave (although some critics may say foolhardy) step and set up her own underground private practice.

Over the course of several years, she treated many patients, together with her husband Konrad, with individual and group psychedelic therapy using LSD, MDMA and 2C-B, until they were arrested and imprisoned. In January 2011, she and Konrad came to stay at my house for a weekend and told me the whole story of those amazing few years. As Friederike recalled:

> Clients would always begin with MDMA. Only when the client was familiar and comfortable with the MDMA experience, sometimes after several individual sessions, would he or she then be invited to join the larger therapeutic psycholytic group. . . . It takes time to get to know and to be with a substance, to recognise the peaks and troughs of it's effects and how to manage one's responses and challenges of the experience.

There is enough data for Friederike to write a whole book on her lifetime's work, which maybe someday she will do. In the meantime, we wrote a paper together, which is due for publication later in 2012 in a forthcoming new journal of the Independent Scientific Committee on Drugs, edited by David Nutt.[43]

Conclusion

As with all research, planning new projects using drugs that have a contentious history needs to be done cautiously to avoid the (often inaccurate) preconceptions about the relative usefulness and harm of these substances. However, common to all these drugs, there exists a rich wealth of anecdotal studies from 40 years ago that were abandoned prematurely before their full therapeutic potential was adequately reported or discounted. This area of psychedelic research is one that provides benefits for furthering our understanding of neuroscience and developing new treatments for our patients. If we are to strive to comprehend the brain in its entirety, these areas are worth revisiting with modern research methods. It is a pleasure to see this happening in so many places throughout the world today.

CHAPTER 10

Psychedelics Caught in the Crossfire of the War on Drugs

"LSD is a psychedelic drug which occasionally causes psychotic behavior in people *who have not taken it*."—Timothy Leary

Crime Pays. War is a Money-spinner. But for Whom?

All wars generate propaganda. It is an effective weapon used on both sides of any debate and we hear a lot of claims about the relative dangers and safety issues in the so-called War on Drugs.

What an extraordinary notion, a war on drugs. It isn't even a war on drug users or drug dealers, but rather a war on the very concept of drugs themselves — well, some drugs, at least, but not alcohol. Could we also wage a war on swearing or a war on nastiness?

Perhaps a more focused war on the *harmful use of drugs* is worth fighting. But increasing numbers of people in our society are now seeing that a prohibition against 98 out of 100 or more psychoactive substances is flawed on so many levels. Whether one approaches the problem from the point of view of health, finance, politics, international crime, class, religion or human rights, it is a war that looks increasingly unwinnable. And if it cannot be won, ought it be fought? And if it is worth fighting, then at what cost, how many resources should be put into it, and how many casualties and how much collateral damage are we prepared to accept?

Many people will say that not only cannot it not be won and ought not be fought, but that it is also a war whose core ideology is rooted in paternalism, religious restriction and even racism and not in the noble sentiments it pretends to uphold. At best, it undoubtedly supports a global crime scene of huge proportions and, at worst, may even *involve* shady government decisions and deals with criminal organisations.

Many people are happy to state that cannabis is the largest cash crop in the United States — more valuable than wheat — but totally unregulated. With no legitimate organisations involved (until the recent medical marijuana cooperatives were established, many of which may now be under threat of closure again) billions of dollars are changing hands without a cent reaching the government purse. For the most part, the drugs industry has no registered companies, no CEOs, no managing directors, no line of responsibility or quality control in place. Instead, criminal gangs whose methods often involve violence and exploitation of vulnerable people shift money from the drug trade around the world.

On the other hand, there is also plenty of evidence that the illegal drugs industry supports many poor people and whole communities of peaceful folk who are otherwise unable to provide for themselves and their families. And when the governments crack down on this cottage industry and attempt to crush the drugs trade, the sufferers are not the rich financiers but the end-game producers and users of the drugs. Meanwhile, the big time suppliers simply drive off in their Mercedes to the next fertile ground for business.

We are told it is a supply-and-demand market perpetuated by the very war itself; it is a war waged against innocent people, ordinary citizens who have committed no other crime than that of having the creativity and enthusiasm to consider experiencing an alternative mental state to their waking consciousness. These innocents are immediately criminalized and forced to dabble in a risky underworld, fraternize with law-breakers and put their careers' and livelihoods at risk.

Those calling for reform of the drug laws will say that the entire hopeless situation could be wiped out at the stroke of pen by the lawmakers. The rug could be pulled from underneath those criminal gangs tomorrow by simply making all drugs legal and available to responsible adults who want them. Those in support of the war, on the other hand, claim such an action would lead to an increase in drug use and an increase in crime and health problems — though it is hard to imagine these issues being very much worse than they are presently. Those in support of legalisation will reply that such a vast sum of money currently goes into prosecuting people through the police, courts and prisons that the savings to be made there would more than adequately free-up funds to transform drug education and treatment services for any possible increase in use that night arise.

A dig at alcohol again: The alcohol lobby is very rich, very much favoured by governments and *very* against seeing other substances compared alongside the risks of booze. They have good reason to worry. It is notable that in 2009 the entire UK NHS budget for providing treatment services for alcohol dependency was the same as the cost of the first six seconds a famous vodka brand's TV commercial. These are the sorts of economics those in favour of encouraging a debate about the evidence-based risks of different substances are up against.

I do not pretend to know enough about the politics and economics of the complex situation surrounding the drug laws to say for certain whose arguments are right in the debate. But as a clinical doctor — and, more critically, as a citizen who has lived through the War on Drugs all my life — I can say with great certainty that after 40 years of successive governments all over the world fighting this campaign what we still seem to have is a massive multi-substance drug problem anywhere one chooses to look. The prisons are full of offenders, trillions are spent on continuing the fight and there is no shortage of new users, new suppliers and — from a clinical point of view — no end in sight of the casualties. Of course, proponents of the war will say these observations are all the more reason while we must keep fighting this war until we win.

There are some excellent organisations pushing tirelessly to encourage debate aimed at reform of the international drug laws.[1] In the UK, we have The Beckley Foundation[2], led by my friend Amanda Feilding, who, alongside sponsoring all manner of consciousness research and psychedelic clinical drug studies, has used her influence in The House of Lords to work with policy makers throughout the world and keep the issue of drug law reforms on the political agenda. (The name of this chapter, incidentally, comes from an article I wrote with Feilding some years ago.)

Evidence-based Decriminalisation and Temple Balls

It is interesting to look at what has been going on in Amsterdam and more recently in Portugal, where legislators have made an evidence-based decision to apply levels of control that are deemed to be more in balance with the actual harms — or harmlessness — of the drugs. Statistics show that since decriminalising cannabis Holland has produced much lower rates of cocaine and heroin use *and* lower rates even of cannabis usage itself per capita than the UK — not to mention lower rates of organised crime, street violence, sexual assaults and teenage pregnancies.[3] Obviously, we cannot relate all these issues to the liberal Dutch approach to cannabis, but what we haven't seen in Holland is the whole country go to pot, as some people here might assume would happen if the UK adopted a similar approach.

When one is presenting lectures on the potential clinical benefits of psychedelic drugs, one frequently gets asked about and drawn into the question of the legalization of drugs for recreational purposes. Personally, I try to keep the two topics as separate as possible, as I see my role primarily as one to advocate for the use of the psychedelic drugs by doctors in a clinical setting. It is often difficult to keep the two issues apart, of course, as I find the errors, inefficiencies and sheer lack of evidence-base for the international drug laws are so stark that they are, as a scientist, almost impossible to ignore.

From a financial point of view, it would seem obvious that legalizing the production of cannabis for the hill farmers of Thailand or other poor communities in the world in Africa and Asia could transform countries like Malawi and Nepal, allowing local communities to finally provide the rest of the world with a unique and sought-after product that only they can make. Imagine that, Malawi Gold and Nepalese Temple Balls (both virtually harmless products, for those without a psychotic fragility) grown as a legitimate cash crop and shipped all over the world to be used by non-law breaking responsible adults everywhere.

MDMA: Are We Throwing the Baby Out with the Bathwater?

But this chapter is not predominantly about the War On Drugs itself but, more specifically, on how it adversely effects medical psychedelic research. A subject I do know a lot about is MDMA and especially how it has been systematically demonised for 23 years in the popular and medical press despite a wealth of evidence for its safe and therapeutic use.[4] 3,4-methylenedioxymethlyamphetamine (MDMA) has penetrated extensively into our culture in the last 30 years. As we have seen, MDMA started life in medicine when adopted as a clinical tool by psychotherapists on the west coast of America who used it as an alternative to the then banned LSD for facilitating interactions in couples' therapy. From the therapist's couch the drug leaked into public use, with a growing recreational use, which eventually led to its prohibition in the mid eighties. As with LSD, the medical research on MDMA then stopped, but its recreational use continued to grow especially in relation to the rave or party scenes so that by the nineties the drug was targeted and loathed by politicians and parents alike.

But while the politicians raved against the drug with a similar ferocity to the kids on the dance floors, the doctors and pharmacologists argued amongst themselves about the short, medium and long term dangers of MDMA. In the background, meanwhile, MDMA as a therapeutic tool was quietly becoming ancient history. Exactly as with LSD before it, the drug had now drifted so far from its clinical origin for this to become forgotten.

But have we missed something important when we allowed the political agenda to hijack MDMA from science and medicine? Has the politicians' single-minded demonization of all recreational drugs as 'Of No Medical Use' resulted in MDMA becoming an innocent bystander caught in the crossfire of the War on Drugs?

Those Evil Blacks and Mexican Drug Users

After all, MDMA is not the first such drug that has been treated in such an unscientific fashion. Cannabis was restricted first in the 1930s and again in the 1950s on the back of blatantly racist campaigns against Mexicans and black Americans, respectively. Indeed, even the name *marijuana* was propagated by the US government of the 1930s because it sounded sufficiently Hispanic to scare off the nice white folks from identifying with those nasty pot-smoking Mexicans. And in the 1950s, the campaign against cannabis was similarly transparently directed at encouraging the same nice white folk to avoid at all costs behaving anything like those crazy jazz-loving, sex-craved blacks. In the UK, on the other hand, where there wasn't such a well-established large non-white community in the 1930s to align with the growing perceived problem of cannabis abuse, the plant has primarily been known simply as cannabis, the valuable source of that durable fabric hemp, and the origin of the word *canvas*. Perhaps this is something some politicians ought to bear in mind next time they are out canvassing support for the war on drugs.

The problem with restricting a drug's recreational use is that it also restricts researching the compound on humans for medical research. And when politics pervades the field of medical research, it threatens to undermine the scientific goals of objectivity that are the cornerstones of practice in the search for evidence-based clinical excellence.[5] MDMA, like cannabis, LSD and psilocybin, could be a useful medical and research tool and all these drugs deserved to be explored in a dispassionate manner without a political agenda influencing the scientific argument.

Just How Dangerous is MDMA?

Whenever a young person dies from a drug-related event involving ecstasy, it tends to make the front page. But the number of column inches occupied by the perceived risks of MDMA is way out of proportion for the actual degree of physical harm that the drug presents and in stark contrast to those frequently occurring as a result of other drugs. Annually in the UK there are around 7000 alcohol-related deaths and 106,000 tobacco-related deaths.[6]

We have heard throughout this book how even the scientific studies exploring the relative harms and safety of MDMA have been misjudged, inaccurate and mislabelled (literally, at times) — all of which add up to a distorted view of the drug in both the scientific and popular opinions. It is difficult to accurately examine the large-scale risks of pure MDMA on human users because most people who take 'ecstasy' (whatever that is) use a host of other drugs too. One interesting study by John Halpern at Harvard looked at neurocognitive functioning in a population of Mormons in the USA who use MDMA *exclusively*, with no lifetime use of any other drugs including alcohol. The results of this study suggest subjects reporting 50 or fewer lifetime episodes of MDMA use displayed no neurocognitive differences approaching significance when compared to non-users.[7]

How Frequently are Clinical Syndromes Attributed to Ecstasy Use?

There are no published studies suggesting psychiatric clinics and wards have become burdened by morbidity due to ecstasy use, which suggests a low incidence of clinical neurotoxicity in human users. Data from a recent neuroimaging study at University College London suggests that MDMA use may not result in long-term damage to serotonin neurons when used recreationally by humans and, furthermore, that when even heavy users stop using the drug within a year there are no demonstrable differences between their brains and brains of people who have never used the drug at all.[8]

Other studies looking at the rates of depression and anxiety among ecstasy users have demonstrated that, when higher levels of depression and anxiety are seen within a group of ecstasy users, this can be related to pre-existing depression and anxiety as children and adolescents, before ever taking ecstasy, emphasising the importance of taking temporal factors into consideration.[9]

The data from retrospective studies measuring functioning in ecstasy users is mixed and there remains a lack of firm conclusions about neurocognitive deficits and psychiatric morbidity. Nevertheless, the debate about the possible dangers of MDMA has had a lot of exposure in both the popular and scientific press in the last 20 years.

Unscientific Attitudes Affecting Medical Research

But the biggest travesty is when popular press media scares are allowed to impact on medical research for exploring a potential clinical role for MDMA as a therapeutic agent to treat mental illness. It is frustrating when scientific studies describing the dangers of taking ecstasy recreationally refer to doses or patterns of use that are irrelevant to the clinical usage of MDMA for psychotherapy. A simple analogy would be to imagine doctors from the Royal College of Surgeons or Anaesthetists being denied access to prescribe, or even *research*, the opiate drugs for clinical use because of the existence of recreational heroin abuse. Opiates are vital parts of these doctors' formulary, and while they are undeniably abused in society, they are also essential clinical tools when used safely by clinicians. MDMA (which is, incidentally, considerably less toxic than the opiates, when used either clinically or recreationally) may have the potential to be an equally important tool for psychiatry.

All these questions make for an interesting proposal that there may be a much larger role for MDMA in clinical medicine than just as an adjunct to psychotherapy. However, with the current drug laws standing as they are, any researcher interested in this field still has significant barriers to overcome before proposing any such projects. Moreover, the controlled status of such compounds in most Western countries deters pharmaceutical companies from even exploring this arena, as they fear that any novel compound with action like MDMA would necessarily be subject to similar legal controls. These would probably hamper its being studied therapeutically and would limit its use and acceptability, even if it were to be shown to have efficacy and to be safer than MDMA in terms of abuse liability, hangover and neurotoxicity.

The Socio-political Agenda on Drugs has a Deleterious Effect on Medical Research

Clinicians, the police, pharmacologists and the general public alike are increasingly questioning the current drug laws. A recent major multidisciplinary review in *The Lancet* by David Nutt and colleagues seriously challenged the current prohibition laws and declared the present system to be not based on scientific foundations.[10] The authors propose that the current system of classification in the UK (in which controlled drugs are classified in classes A, B and C) does not always accurately reflect the true physical harm, risk of dependence and social harm of controlled drugs. They used delphic analysis to more accurately classify twenty potential drugs of abuse — including legal drugs such as alcohol and tobacco — into a hierarchy. This form of analysis utilises a lengthy and broad discussion by experts in multiple fields using principles of evidence-based medicine to more precisely assess the drug's potential for harm. The results suggest there is no significant correlation between the current Misuse of Drugs Act and the harm rating elicited by this analytical method. While some drugs currently classified as the most harmful (Class A) also scored highly in the Lancet study (for example, heroin and cocaine), other drugs that are currently Class A, such as ecstasy and LSD scored very low in the harm rating. And conversely, some of the legal drugs (alcohol, tobacco and benzodiazepines) scored highly. A system that allows for drugs such as alcohol and nicotine to be freely available while drugs with less damaging pharmacological profiles are criminalised is bound to give off the wrong message to the public.

The Lancet paper demonstrates that our current methods for assessing harm are not based on the most accurate medical or social evidence but on other, unscientifically-motivated socio-political factors. In the 1960s, a similar association between psychedelic drug use and the undesirable left-wing politics that challenged the authorities over foreign policy in Vietnam was often quoted in debates that lead to the eventual prohibition of LSD in 1966.

David Nutt proposed the laws be changed to reflect the actual harms of the drugs and in particular suggested that:

i.   MDMA go from Class A to Class B
ii. LSD from Class A to Class B
iii. Cannabis from Class B to Class C

But he was controversially sacked by the Labour government of the day for his opinions. He made some erudite — but clearly annoying for the authorities — comments. Outraged at the government disregarding the clear objective advice of experts in the field in favour of their preconceived political agenda he, perhaps in retrospect, overstepped the mark and openly criticised the government's policies. But he has lost no favour from the scientific community since that decision — far from it. Okay, so those supporting the Labour (and Conservative) policies of total prohibition may consider him a lose cannon and a maverick, but this is not at all tangible in the scientific community, where he remains as respected as ever — if not more so, for his courage.

Having split from the ACMD, Nutt formed a new committee in 2010 called the Independent Scientific Committee On Drugs (ISCD), which is not, as the name suggests, a group of intoxicated independent scientists but, rather, an attempt to gather and disseminate scientific research in an unbiased fashion without the influence of politicians putting their own spin on the data.[11]

Medical Research with Psychedelics Requires Courage

The development of MDMA as a tool to assist psychotherapy is now well underway, but perhaps the next stage of exploring the drug's potential lies in proposing a study that investigates it's role as a potent serotonin agonist to rapidly elevate mood. However, a study such as this remains extremely difficult to put forward given the continuing prohibition. Should such studies prove successful they could offer a novel approach to the treatment of depression although the current laws mitigate against pharmaceutical companies following up such findings with new drugs with the same actions. This situation is bad for science and bad for patients and quite illogical. We must not let MDMA research be hijacked by politics, as has happened with LSD. MDMA is a medical tool and it deserves to remain within medicine.

While it is clearly beyond the scope of this book to challenge such ingrained political dogmas as the international War On Drugs, what I can hope to do is encourage and support a technocratic approach to the drug laws, especially in regard to how they impact on psychiatric drug research.

It will take a brave politician to finally come off the fence and use the clear evidence wisely to review the archaic drug laws. But in reward for this bravery, that politician would be instantly popular and remembered historically for his or her good sense. That moment in history might still be some way off, although when the time comes it will come suddenly. The balance will tip with alarming speed once the politicians of the world realise they are freed from the senseless moral and twisted ethical constraints that keep the prohibition going. This is what political commentators call 'the seat belt effect' — that moment when, after years of intense resistance and debate, the arguments suddenly stop. It is now globally accepted that by all that seat belts must be worn in cars, and we wonder now why there was ever a problem about it in the first place. The drugs debate could go the same way.

In the meantime, we can hope that medicine, at least, if not the world's safe and diligent users of psychedelic drugs, can be freed up to choose whichever mental states they wish to indulge in the safety and privacy of their own minds.

The Concept of Harm Minimisation

In 1998 the organisation DanceSafe was formed to provide information at raves and offer ecstasy users a service for testing the quality of the pills they were taking in order to reduce casualties associated with low quality and adulterated substances.[12] But the concept of safe raving is much older than that. Since the sixties, festivals have included 'trip tents' where stressed-out users can go for psychological support or medical treatment. One such current organisation is Kosmicare, which provides excellent support for ravers at festivals throughout Europe.[13]

When I worked at the Glastonbury festival for six years in the medical tent as one of the resident psychiatrists, our main role was being with and seeing people through difficult drug experiences. Rarely were people in any significant physical harm — except for the ones who had drunk too much alcohol, they were always considered the most risky. Those who had taken psychedelic drugs and were having a hard time because of their lack of attention to set and setting often presented as scared and lost in strange surroundings having become separated from their friends. All that was needed most of the time was few hours chatting to our team and a cup of tea, and then they'd be on their way again. My friend Karin Silenzi de Stagni, however, the director and founder of Kosmicare, offers a more thorough approach to bewildered trippers, delivered by a skilled team of experienced psychonauts This is an important service for those who have become existentially separated from their buddies and their bodies.

In the late 1980s, when the concept of looking after ravers became established in the UK, there was outrage from right-wing groups. I remember talking to people at raves in the early 1990s that were campaigning for clubs to give out free drinking water and provide chill out rooms for over-heated ravers. Critics argued that such measures were condoning ecstasy use. But all these groups wanted to do was to save lives and reduce harm.

It is ironic that now, some 25 years later, the modern NHS has embraced the concept of harm minimisation, rightly choosing it over total prohibition as the most appropriate and safe evidence-based approach to reducing the harms of casual drug use. Thankfully, those working with substance misuse disorders have been successful at convincing the authorities that people are going to continue to take drugs, whether the politicians like it or not, so measures that reduce the harm of such behaviours ought to be employed. A really stark illustration of just how far harm minimisation has come in the last 20 years can be found in the wealth of government leaflets and information available to today's drug users. I have seen NHS government-sanctioned cartoons aimed at children encouraging them to 'chase the dragon' rather than inject heroin, and I recently saw an interesting government leaflet on crack cocaine. It used a series of cartoons to advice the user to pay their rent and buy their week's groceries before going out and scoring their crack with their Job Seekers Allowance money. Then it recommended that, when coming to the last rock of the day, take time to savour and enjoy it, as there would be no more until tomorrow! It may sound crazy for those who would like to just say no to drugs, but the reality is this kind of advice does reduce harm and save lives and there is no evidence to suggest it makes people want to go out and actually *start* taking crack if they hadn't been inclined to do so in the first instant.[14]

But there are still right-wing voices closing down needle exchanges. And David Nutt recently reiterated the call for pill testing in clubs but certainly did not get a lot positive support from everyone. Harm minimisation saves lives and people always have and always will take substances to alter their state of consciousness. It is the job of doctors and politicians to reduce harm, not try to deny or eradicate the urges of consenting adults who wish to indulge in relatively harmless activities.

Demonization of Prohibition

It is interesting that the word *prohibition* is increasingly being used in reference to the War on Drugs. The term *prohibition* is universally accepted as a political bad idea, a failed attempt to enforce an un-enforceable law against alcohol. It is widely recognised that the prohibition of the 1930s directly fuelled the development of the mafia-driven criminal networks. Perhaps we are seeing some positive steps towards enlightenment today as regards all illicit drugs? I doubt it, but it would not be before time if we were.

Perhaps one day we will look back on the War on Drugs and laugh in the same way as we do about the 1930s experiment. All those wasted years, money and lives. The War On Drugs, waged by successive governments against all substances with abuse potential, threatens to strangle our advancement of knowledge about how these substances might be used safely and effectively to treat patients with unremitting mental illnesses. We do not seek to condone the recreational use of potentially dangerous compounds, but, rather, to view the subject with a scientific objectivity that the political agenda is often seen to be lacking. Such an approach is essential if we are to provide the most effective and targeted social policies around prohibition and, crucially, the best evidenced treatments for our patients.

Why Does This Issue Matter?

There are dangers associated with inaccurately reporting an exaggerated risk of drug use in the scientific and popular press. It may provoke a public health scare resulting in disproportionate use of resources and money, which could be better directed elsewhere and it risks directing attention and education away from more effective harm-minimisation programs. But perhaps the most important side effect of inaccurate reporting is the damage it inflicts to research exploring potential positive therapeutic benefits of the drug.

No attempt is being made to condone recreational drug use or suggest that MDMA or any other illegal substance is an entirely safe drug; after all, there is no such thing. There are valid concerns that MDMA, for instance, can induce low mood as its effects wear off, that it can induce pre-existing anxiety and depression in susceptible individuals, that it produces unwanted acute side-effects such as spasmodic contractions of the jaw muscles and that in very rare cases of uncontrolled recreational use it can cause an idiosyncratic adverse reaction that may even be fatal. But for all drugs, whether used recreationally or prescribed, the public deserve to be given a realistic risk-benefit ratio and accurate reporting of relative risks as they apply to them.

A lot of water has passed under the bridge since ecstasy emerged as a potential problem in 1988 and since then an abundance of studies have not confirmed irreversible neurotoxicity in humans or an associated rise in clinical morbidity from the use of MDMA.

The table below, by Gable, gives a nice picture of where some of the psychedelic drugs lie in a table charting abuse potential (addictive risk) and lethal dose.[15] Drugs in the top right hand corner are the most dangerous and those in the lower left hand corner are the safest. Note how the placement of the drugs in this table is in such stark contrast to their current legal status. In my opinion as a doctor, it is nicotine's place on this table that is by far the most worrying feature. Heroin and cocaine we all know about, but nicotine and alcohol are available for sale outside every school on every street corner. Weird.

Recreational Drug Use for Psycho-spiritual Growth

Before this current renaissance got underway, Albert Hofmann famously said that next time psychedelic drugs enjoy a resurgence in society 'the medical doctors

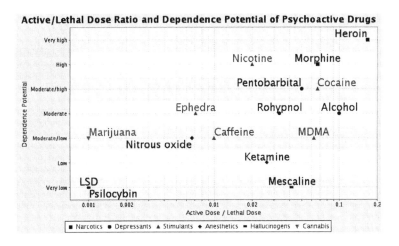

must not be allowed to run the show'. Earlier, I made the statement earlier that as a clinical doctor campaigning for the medical use of psychedelic drugs (as opposed to commenting on the recreational use of drugs), I must not allow myself to be dragged into the debate about whether non-clinical populations ought to be able to use the psychedelics. I am nevertheless now going to contradict myself. This is because I do believe there are some circumstances in which healthy, non-clinical members of society can use these currently illegal drugs safely. Drugs such as LSD, psilocybin, cannabis and MDMA *can* be used carefully, with adequate preparation by an individual to enrich their life. These substances can provide valuable insights and opportunities for reflection, especially as regards important personal existential issues and issues to do with their relationships with others.

I therefore support those lobbies of sensible, non-hedonistic users who choose to push for legalisation of drugs to be used judiciously for such positive uses. Hofmann hoped that one day his discovery, LSD, might become available legally, to be used in clinics where people can safely connect with one another and with nature in a facilitative environment. In effect, such places do exist already in the form of those religious organisations that use substances legitimately, such as the Santo Daime and União do Vegetal Church's use of ayahuasca, the West African use of ibogaine and the Native American Church's use of peyote.

But why not imagine a day where psychedelics can be used in a Western context? American writer and psychedelic researcher Thomas Roberts has done just this and presents wonderful talks about his vision for a one-billion-dollar company, Community Psychedelic Centers International, which will provide education, training and opportunities for psychedelic voyages on the high street from registered premises.[16] His book *Psychedelic Horizons* is a marvellous piece of writing that avoids the clichéd backstory of psychedelic history and looks firmly towards the future.[17]

The psychedelic journey is a deeply personal and profoundly important experience. To deny a healthy and functioning person such a unique existential experience is bordering on a restriction of fundamental human rights. And while these substances are not, in any shape or form, a panacea to cure all ills, there is good anecdotal evidence — from millions of users worldwide — that through the careful use of such drugs one can not only transform for the better one's personal life but this can have a positive effect on one's immediate environment by providing a space for community reflection. These are not tested suppositions, because of the ban on such widespread use of these drugs, but this is potentially valuable area of study that deserves its place in the future of psychedelic research.

In Conclusion

There are many people battling for governments all over the world to look with sense at the drug laws for all kinds of reasons: from those wishing for medical research to progress unhindered by irritating regulatory processes to those simply wanting the religious freedom to choose to alter their mental state in whatever way they see fit within the safe confines of their own home.

But a major problem with the fight against the War On Drugs is that there are wildly different methodological arguments being used on either side of the debate. On the one side, there are the likes of David Nutt and the Beckley Foundation producing reams of accurate objective data supporting an end to prohibition. But, on the other side, are governments whose agenda is influenced by the powerful drinks industry and a right-wing media fuelled not by science but by a conservative sentimental approach. Being seen to be 'soft on drugs' is a known vote loser. But just because the general masses are scared of a position that offers radical changes to the current system does not mean the current position is right. One despairs sometimes and wonders just how much more scientific or sociological data will it take before the blinkered politicians take notice.

Clearly, as Thomas Roberts says, rather than sitting back and waiting for our esteemed leaders to become enlightened with a natural urge to embrace transpersonal issues, the answer instead is to meet the business people and the politicians (they are the same thing) head on with the kind of argument they can understand: votes and money. If the culture can be shifted towards an accurate assessment of the risks then the general public will support whatever brave politician dares to put their head above the parapet and propose a reform of the drug laws. And as soon as the politicians realise that in doing so there is an awful lot of money to made — and saved — by providing drugs to those who want them, and treatment for those that need it, then the seeds of change will be sown very quickly indeed. Until then we will just have to wait. The current situation certainly gives a lot of people a career. One thing is for sure, there is no way I would be writing this book if I had chosen to study the research of non-psychoactive, politically benign heart tablets.

Conclusion

Back to the Future

Psychiatry Needs Psychedelics, and Psychedelics Need Psychiatry

Without researching these drugs for medical therapy, psychiatry is turning its back on a group of compounds that could have great potential. Without the validation of the medical profession, the psychedelic drugs will remain archaic vestiges of the past, maligned as recreational drugs of abuse and subject to continued negative opinion. Similarly, the people who use them — even for psycho-spiritual purposes — will remain maligned and rejected by society.

These two disparate groups — psychiatrists and recreational psychedelic drug users — are united by their shared recognition of the healing potential of these compounds. Progression for both groups will come from professionals working in the field adapting to fit a conservative paradigm. This way they can provide the public with important treatments and also raise the profile of expanded consciousness in mainstream society.

The spring 2011 Breaking Convention Conference in Canterbury, UK was the first British conference dedicated entirely to psychedelics, and it was important that the medical profession was adequately represented. Psychedelic drugs have had a consistent presence in the UK since the 1960s, as both a hedonistic recreational pursuit and as part of a creative subculture, while their clinical use has regrettably fallen from the medical curriculum for the last forty years. But recently, we have seen a re-emergence of these compounds in medicine. They have re-entered the mainstream with impressive force, pushing them to the forefront of contemporary brain research.

But what about the hippies? The interplay between psychiatry and psychedelia has been part of the necessary developmental trajectory for our culture and we can now see a new way — a renaissance as some are calling it — initiating a reformation of the relationship between the people using these drugs, their society, science and greater spiritual consciousness. This is the future. We are going back to it.

Prehistoric and Recent Psychotherapy with Psychedelics

As we have seen in this book, the ancient use of hallucinogens for the augmentation of psychotherapy is well documented by scholars of anthropology. All cultures through history have used sacramental plants and fungi to assist individuals and communities access repressed memories. The role of shamans, with their combined roles of physicians, psychotherapists and priests, and the nature of their relationship with their patients, is not dissimilar to that of the today's psychotherapists.

The rediscovery of the healing aspects of psychedelics between the 1940s and 1970s was set to become the next big thing in psychiatry. Before that, psychiatrists were restricted largely to psychoanalytical methods crudely augmented by imprecise physical treatments such as insulin coma therapy, psychosurgery and un-anesthetised electroconvulsive therapy.

In the 1950s, there was an explosion of interest in newly emerging psychotropic drugs such as the phenothiazines, which whetted the appetites of psychiatrists looking for a pharmacological solution for their patients' disorders. It is against this background that Hofmann's Delysid ushered in the world's first large-scale use of psychedelic therapy on psychiatric patients. LSD shone the light on the archaic uses of psychedelics, and, in the 1950s, spawned a global interest in the cross-cultural dimension of hallucinogens.

Now, after some 40 years of repressive actions of successive governments to effectively halt all psychedelic research (while the recreational use of every other drug has increased tenfold), we are seeing a growth of contemporary psychedelic research. Numerous clinical and neurophysiological studies are being published every week. The expansive growth of our understanding of the physiological processes behind the subjective psychological effects of psychedelic drugs is informed hugely by imaging techniques. This provides an envious perspective from which to re-visit studies of the 1950s and 1960s. Back then, we had to simply take it for granted that these substances 'increased access to repressed emotional memories'. Now we can demonstrate this graphically with cutting edge neuroimaging, which adds kudos to the field and courts greater interest from those mainstream-funding organisations that previously considered psychedelic research to be of the archaic past.

The Problem with Psychiatry

But despite advances in research methods, psychiatry remains the Cinderella of the medical profession. Even as modern brain studies narrow the gap between the dated concepts of 'functional' versus 'organic' mental illness, today's psychiatrists remain decades behind our general medical cousins in our understanding of the body's most challenging organ. This is not surprising given the brain's complexity. There are a hundred-billion neurons in the human brain connected to one another by up to ten-thousand dendrites per neuron. A single cubic millimetre of grey matter contains over three kilometres of axons. These are staggering statistics that makes organs such as the liver, kidney and heart seem crudely simple by comparison.

However, we do not have to go far back in medical history to find an age when physicians were equally baffled by the physical body. 150 years ago medicine had a good idea about the epidemiology of many common diseases. We could accurately describe who got smallpox, which populations were at risk of infections and what was happening at a gross anatomical level. Nineteenth-century doctors voluminously categorised the diseases they saw and mapped their progressions through populations. But they had little idea about the pathophysiological nature of these common disorders and, crucially, they could not see a way to actually treat them. However, just around the corner was a critical advance, the antibiotics, and once discovered the face of mortality statistics were changed forever.

Today the psychiatric profession is in a similar position to those nineteenth century physicians. We enthusiastically categorise and track the epidemiology of psychiatric disorders, writing thick diagnostic manuals to describe who gets anxiety and depression and how childhood maltreatment effects future mental health. But we still lack agreement on effective treatments and continue to ask: *Where is our psychiatric antibiotic?* At best, contemporary treatments partially mask the symptoms of mental disorder. Antidepressant drugs may help a person to appear broadly happier and retain some degree of functioning. But these crude treatments do not get to the heart of the problem. They do not provide a 'psychic antibiotic' to get in under the skin of the person's traumatic past and attack the lesion at its source.

The research and pharmaceutical industries are not adequately challenging this status quo. Indeed, some organisations thrive on drug treatments that require a daily dose of their expensive product, to be taken indefinitely and with a transparent realisation that it will never actually 'cure' them of their problem. Of course, as doctors we support the pharmaceutical industry and readily prescribe their drugs –– we have to — they are all we have. It would be unethical *not* to mask the symptoms of psychiatric disorder for those patients. But we know the drugs we give are often not doing anything to resolve their problem. It feels as if nothing short of returning the desperate patients to the psychological scenes of their youth so they live out and resolve their issues in real waking time will be effective at helping them exorcise those demons. But what possible psychiatric treatment could provide that kind of effect?

Why Psychedelic Medicine Works

Psychedelics are the perfect drugs to assist psychotherapy. They are short-acting so can be administered for a single session of therapy. They have no significant dependency issues. They are completely non-toxic at doses proposed for therapy (and are considerably safer than the medications we currently use in psychiatry). They are shown to reduce depression. They raise arousal to enhance motivation for therapy, increase feelings of closeness between the patient and therapist, increase relaxation and reduce hypervigilance. They stimulate new ways of thinking to explore entrenched problems. And drugs such as MDMA also have the important characteristic of being able to *reduce the fear of recalling of traumatic memories* so the patient can focus intensely on their trauma without being overwhelmed by negative feelings. When the pharmacological effects of psychedelic drugs are combined with effective and expertly guided psychotherapy they can offer a new way of looking at old psychiatric problems and could just be the Holy Grail, the penicillin just around the corner for psychiatry.

Using the guided psychedelic experience as medicine, we can tentatively allow ourselves to use a forbidden word, a word that as medical students on our first psychiatric placement we are conditioned never to utter. It is the word *cure*. With psychedelic drug therapy we *can* turn back time, return to face miserable childhood memories, back to the child's bedroom where that horrific abuse occurred and, psychologically at least, *rewrite history* for that patient. Under the influence of drugs such as MDMA, LSD, ayahuasca and psilocybin — used with care and supervision — these patients can in real, waking time stare into the face of their memories of abuse, explore and repackage the sensory aspects of those recollections and *put that memory away* in the compartmentalized area of their past where it belongs. The memory will always be there; the psychedelic drugs will not simply nullify or blunt out history (we leave that to the toxic effects of the traditional prescribed psychotropics and drugs like heroin and alcohol), but psychedelics can help patients re-label their past experiences and become masters of their minds, not remain slaves to the random emergence of unwanted memories that blight their waking and sleeping lives. This unique and powerful role of the psychedelic drugs is tailor-made for disorders based around anxiety. And these disorders are not rare. Anxiety, including PTSD and OCD, are the scourge of modern psychiatry, the smallpox and gangrene of our modern age.

But above these clinically useful effects of the psychedelic drugs there is something else — a mysterious, apparently *spiritual* element that defies our current medical language. The existential component of the psychedelic experience is undeniable and is why these compounds are so useful for improving the resolution of end-of-life anxiety. But the subject of psychedelic spirituality, while wholeheartedly embraced by the recreational users of these drugs, sits uncomfortably with most medical doctors. It was this spiritual element — and the hippies love of it — that blew the opportunity for medical psychedelic research in the past. This time round we need to be slightly more cautious.

The Problem with the Recreational Use of Psychedelics

When LSD was banned in the mid sixties, medical research was severely limited worldwide. Illegalisation had a paradoxical effect on restricting popular use, subsequently producing the massive 1960s drug culture. Young people embraced LSD and cannabis, popularly accepted as a rite of passage, a de rigour ticket to the swirling maelstrom of anti-authoritarianism left-wing protest and the rejection of the older generation. LSD became labelled as a drug to enhance creativity and was highly influential in colouring new approaches to multiple disciplines from art, music and architecture to fashion, product design, TV and film production and even cooking. Indeed, never before in human history had so many people been so influenced by such a small molecule.

Inevitably, this revolution irked those in authority whose grip on power was threatened by a group of people whose *raison d'etre* was to encourage freedom of thought beyond the preceding necessarily restricted modes of expression. Doctors, when banned from research with the drug except under very constrained circumstances, were forced to further distance themselves from using LSD with their patients and instead had to toe the party line. What had started as a legitimate and effective new line of psychiatric research was now driven underground. This was disheartening for those clinicians who had seen how useful psychedelic therapy was for patients where traditional methods had failed. Most gave up their research with psychedelics and returned to mainstream medicine, embracing the growing arsenal of new symptom-masking psychotropic chemicals flooding the market, fuelled by pharmaceutical corporations eager to cash in on the physical approach to treating mental disorders, which, ironically, was begun in part by the interest in LSD fifteen years earlier. Later on, some of the early medical psychedelic pioneers turned their attention to the then-still-legal drug MDMA and developed systems for its use in psychotherapy until it too was banned in the 1980s and, following a broadly similar path to LSD, created the nineties rave generation.

Having lost the medical profession as allies, the late-sixties hippies were now free to become the mouthpiece of the psychedelic revolution. Building their churches and laboratories in the free festivals and communal living, they propagated their philosophy and re-wrote the political codes and boundaries of the New Age, combining the utopian dream of sham political organisation alongside the contradictory banner of boundary-free living, as informed by the ego-less freedom of the internal hallucinatory world. And when mainstream pop society came down from the 1960s and turned back to the grindstone of consumer-driven modern living, those brave pioneers still willing to fly the freak flag, as it were, became increasingly maligned. Their message of internal freedom fell on deaf ears for the majority of clean-living (alcohol soaked) people.

The drugs themselves had moved on. The beautiful people of Haight-Ashbury had morphed into a homeless army of amphetamine and heroin addled ghosts. What had started out as a legitimate protest to an unwinnable foreign war in Vietnam now looked to many like senseless disturbance of the peace. The message was drugs are bad. Drugs ruin lives. Drugs are used only by directionless scroungers. Without the considered approach from the medical profession adding a level of evidence-based caution to the use of psychedelics as medicines, the hippies' message was lost. Gone were the academics preaching a careful methodological approach. All that was left was 'getting kicks'.

Of course, there always have been some pockets of well-organised users advocating a considered method of using psychedelic drugs as healing agents, but these were few and far between. The subsequent developing cocaine trade further restricted any honourable or noble message of the dying hippies and LSD was lost in the mire. The 1960s didn't work. Drug-crazed hippies don't think straight — why should they? By their very definition, their drugs cause an 'acute confusional state' and don't sit well with complex messages about re-evaluation of social values. The 'normal' people had already concluded that it was exactly these drugs that had caused society's problems in the first place.

Doctors, politicians and the other grey-suited 'men of wisdom' have always struggled with groups of long-haired soothsayers whose sentences end with the word 'man'. Glastonbury's stone circle and Burning Man — wonderful, beautiful, creative, life-affirming, progressive and spiritually awakened social melting pot experiments that they are — do not sit well within the austere chambers of the Royal Medical Colleges, or Westminster. In these places the hair is neatly trimmed and the shirts well-pressed. It is arguable that such stolid attitudes need to be challenged — and, indeed, many before and since Leary have tried, but none have been successful.

Doctors and indeed politicians need randomised double-blind placebo controlled clinical studies, not reports of anecdotal drug experiences, no matter how convincing they may seem to the saucer-eyed users. Until recently, the medical profession had no choice but to reject the hippies and join forces with the politicians. They did their bit for the War on Drugs by churning out studies highlighting the dangers of wanton recreational use of substances. Forced to appraise individuals' mental breakdowns in the context of their drug use, they categorised illegal drugs as agents that solely cause harm. By the time we saw ecstasy step up to take LSD's place of 'killer drug' in the early nineties, neurocognitive deficits and brain damage were the phrases of the day. Doctors and neuroscientists wrote voraciously, applying endless erroneous assumptions about doses and patterns of use of recreational ecstasy users, forgetting that one man's cognitive impairment was another man's party. The medical profession, proudly contributing to the entrenched position of the system, pitched itself against the ravers in the same manner as they had become accustomed to attacking the hippies. The War on Drugs had stepped up a gear and The Man had won.

The Problem with the Medical Use of Psychedelics

But medicine does not have all the answers. Randomised controlled trials (RCTs), although the gold standard of research, the benchmark for all new treatments, are highly artificial phenomena. Psychedelic psychotherapy has never sat comfortably with RCTs. How do you design a reliable psychotherapy placebo? And how do you double-blind an experience as intensely *known* as high-dose LSD? But these are not the major hurdles to hallucinogen research. The main challenge lies in convincing a profession funded by the pharmaceutical industry to spend millions on researching and developing a therapy that could end up challenging the need for antidepressants.

Who normally pays for (non-psychedelic) psychotherapy? The couch makers? The truth is they rarely get done. Large-scale randomised, controlled trials of psychotherapy, difficult to design and expensive to run, are few and far between. It would be nice to imagine the pharmaceutical companies have patients' best interests at heart, that they wish to nobly pursue an programme that aims to wipe out mental disorder altogether, but control, not cure, is their agenda. And without the financial support of multi-million companies encouraging the media (and therefore public) to look at psychedelics, the press is free to propagate whatever message it wants. Money dictates medical research. Doctors and researchers do not want to bite the hand that feeds them, no matter how subtly that food is supplied.

The delay by the medical profession to develop a consistent evidence-based approach to the relative harms and safety of recreational drugs with coincidental therapeutic potential has been continually hampered by a negative media profile. Psychedelic drugs are not *entirely* safe — no drug or indeed any medical intervention is — but, statistically, they are *very* safe. And now, over 20 years since 1988's Summer of Love, we are starting to get a balanced opinion in the press. Indeed, it is now only the lone voices of non-clinical opponents, with limited experience of the plight of patients, that are unable to appreciate that psychedelic therapy bears little resemblance to unrestrained recreational use. The popular belief that 'All Recreational Drugs Kill' is no longer a valid argument against the low to moderate infrequent doses of psychedelics applied as medical treatments.

But we certainly didn't get here through the efforts of the ravers or the hippies. Most of their mental twittering of the last forty years has been ignored by mainstream society. It was only through the more recent and considered change in direction of hard-nosed scientists that we are seeing this so-called renaissance. Sadly, by watering down the mystical-spiritual elements of psychedelics, today's researchers have got their work underway. Even Roland Griffith's tremendous piece of scientific art, which is a point in case, uses a necessarily conservative language with which to disseminate his important message to his doubting medical colleagues. And all of us working in psychedelic research know that it is essential to downplay the more 'cosmic' components of our work in order to get funding and publication. It is only through developing a language of conservative banality that we are where we are today.

This is not a satisfactory position. Why should doctors not use words like *bliss* and *enlightenment*? Psychiatry is overly restricted and restrictive in describing mental states only in a language of pathology. The medical model is insufficient to accurately portray what it is to soar angelic on psychedelic drugs. By avoiding descriptions of the psychedelic experience in its glorious entirety, because of impositions from the bodies that fund the research, we risk missing the transpersonal and not eking from these drugs the full extent of their offering. By taking a polarised swing to the extreme of the hippies' standpoint, the medical profession may be missing the wood for the trees and developing substandard therapy paradigms that fail to incorporate the essential healing elements of the naturalistic psychedelic experience. The hippies, of course, have no qualms about including as much cosmic language as they can muster.

While a legitimate mainstream license to practice for MDMA psychotherapy for PTSD might be only a decade away, it is hard to imagine that NHS doctors will be embracing the full cross-cultural practice of South American ayahuasca use in the near future or that in-the-field ibogaine therapy will be delivered by West Africans in dreary NHS clinics any time soon. It seems the little white pills will be given out long before Western doctors become comfortable prescribing night-long sessions with painted-faced shamans.

Does this matter? Yes it does. Psychedelic psychotherapy, if it is to be effective, must embrace the full healing element of the experience; a watered down capsulated version will not suffice. Furthermore, by conforming to such restrictions the medical profession risks further polarising these drugs into those that are acceptable and those that are not. We would continue to operate on an uneven playing field. All healing substances used by all healers ought to have an equal footing in medicine. Doctors may still have something to learn from the hippies.

Resolution of These Problems

We need to introduce these drugs gently. By working within the necessarily restricting guidelines of mainstream methodological practice, we can hope to avoid giving our influential press-writers any excuse to align the hedonistic recreational use of non-psychedelic, more destructive drugs with the sober intentions of the medical psychedelic community. Boring, I know, but essential. Like it or not, we need to appeal to the sensibilities of the herd.

But it's not just conservatives who need convincing. There are still many doubters of the healing effects of psychedelic drugs within the medical profession itself. We must get these people on our side now alongside persuading the general public. Doctors must infiltrate their medical journals with case studies, book reviews and well-designed studies so cynics can understand that the psychedelic projects of recent years are some of the most eloquent psychopharmacology studies around. The recent projects have had to be of the highest quality, with critics intensely vigilant and ready to strike at the first hint of methodological limitation.

We need a new language with which to talk about the psychedelic experience and perhaps even (sorry Aldous and Humphrey) a new name for these compounds. *Psycholytic*, *entheogen* or *entactogen* are all viable alternatives to the now too negatively biased *psychedelic*. These substances are not recreational drugs, they are medical agents, pharmacological compounds designed in the main part in laboratories by and for the medical profession. That is where they started and that is where they deserve to return. We owe that much to the population of patients with intractable mental health disorders who may benefit from their effects.

Having been woefully absent from our education since the 1970s, the psychedelic drugs need to be bought back in to mainstream university teaching as viable medicines to treat a range of mental disorders. Negative attitudes to novel approaches often develop at medical school and then persist throughout the profession. Scholars must use creative techniques to bring psychedelic culture to the attention of new generations of psychiatrists.

We must overcome the medical model and embrace the mental states of bliss, enlightenment and spiritual emergence. These are valid *mental states* experienced by many people. That they are difficult to comprehend and describe with our current medical language does not mean they do not exist, any more than suggesting the mental state of *love* doesn't exist, just because we find it difficult to describe with psychiatric language. The states of bliss and enlightenment have been the prime possession of the world's religions for too long. But why should they own them? These are *mental states*, with the same empirical validity as depression, anxiety and agitation — all perfectly recognised by psychiatrists. It is time for psychiatrists to wrestle these words back off religions and embrace them within the sphere of medicine.

The economics of psychedelic medicine are also convincing once understood. Effective psychotherapy augmented by psychedelics is a cost-effective way of treating otherwise unremitting mental illnesses. If, as the emerging evidence suggests, a few focused drug-assisted sessions with MDMA or psilocybin can truly eliminate the symptoms of chronic mental disorders *for good*, then this means the patient need not continue with lengthy and expensive pharmacological treatments and the immense financial and personal burden of psychiatric disease on the community can be reduced. Doctors, politicians and the general public alike will embrace any new approach that can effectively demonstrate such a phenomenon. Psychedelic therapy clinics could become commonplace in our communities. In the future, psychedelic drugs need not be confined only to clinical populations but could be made available to much larger groups of healthy people. They could use these substances under appropriate supervision in licensed premises for their own personal psycho-spiritual growth and development. Why not?

Summary of this Book and Orientation for Future Direction

We need to forget trying to change our pseudo-apocalyptical world and the course of human history with psychedelics as they did in the 1960s. Such arrogance is beyond reason in the twenty-first century when society is far too varied for such a restricted viewpoint. Everything possible must be done to avoid the past promises of chemical utopia. Indeed, an unfortunate but necessary truth is that professionals working in this field must remain as boring and staid as possible — as well as inspirational and enthusiastic — to get the message across.

To finish, and by way of a disclaimer, I do not say all of these dull and conservative things because I lack imagination or fail to appreciate the fun, wonder and spirituality of the psychedelic experience. On the contrary, I welcome and embrace it. But I firmly believe that those of us who see the benefits of psychedelic drugs have a much better chance of infiltrating our message into mainstream consciousness if we adopt a cautious approach. And the net result is that this way we may eventually get psychedelic psychotherapy in through the back door.

Then we really will have a revolution, man.

Acknowledgments

Thank you to Mark Chaloner and that long-time inspirer of the less tangible, Tim Read, at Muswell Hill Press for their support and for giving me the opportunity to express in words with virtually unchecked passion what I have carried around in my head for so long.

I am grateful to Keiron Le Grice for reviewing the manuscript and providing not only prose-perfect editing, and feedback based on a knowledge of the subject, but also providing me with appropriate boundaries and helping me keep my feet on the ground while allowing my head to remain in the clouds. And, similarly, thanks again to Leaf Fielding whose comments and support are appreciated.

Special thanks to go Dave and Rick for the forewords and the years of inspirational encouragement that have helped me keep going and ignore the harbingers of doom with their comments of 'career suicide'. But most of all thank you to my clever and beautiful wife Sarah for enduring this process and believing in me, even if not always believing me. Look! It's finished — I'm back!

B.S.
June 2012

Notes

Introduction

1. The song 'The Half Remarkable Question', by The Incredible String Band from the album *Wee Tam and The Big Huge*. This band's music is an excellent place to start for anyone interested in what the psychedelic experience sounds like.
2. Timothy Leary offers these words on his album of speech and psychedelic music from 1967, *Turn On Tune In Drop Out*.
3. McKenna, Terence (1982) *Food of the Gods*. London: Bantam.

Chapter 1: A Personal Reflection

1. Strassman, Rick (1995) *DMT: The Spirit Molecule*. New York: Park Street Press.
2. www.maps.org
3. Sandison, R. and Sessa, B. (2008) 'An Interview with Dr Ronald Sandison – LSD Pioneer in UK Psychiatry'. *Multidisciplinary Association for Psychedelic Studies Bulletin.* Autumn Volume, 2008.
4. www.beckleyfoundation.org
5. Sessa, Ben (2005) 'Can psychedelics have a role in psychiatry again?' *British Journal of Psychiatry 186*: 457–458.
6. Sessa, Ben (2006) 'Psychosis, Psychedelics and the Transpersonal Journey': Proceedings of the Royal College of Psychiatrists Spirituality and Psychiatry Special Interest Group Programme for Friday 31st March, 2006.
7. Nutt, David J. et al (2007) 'The Development of a rational scale to assess the harm of drugs of potential misuse'. *The Lancet*, vol. 369: 1047–1053.
8. Home Office (2009) 'MDMA ('ecstasy'): A review of its harms and classification under the Misuse of Drugs Act 1971.' http://www.erowid.org/chemicals/mdma/mdma_info13.pdf
9. A copy of the letter from Labour government Home Secretary, Alan Johnson, to David Nutt can be found here: http://www.bbc.co.uk/blogs/thereporters/markeaston/2009/10/nutt_gets_the_sack.html
10. Carhart-Harris, Robin L.; Williams, Tim M.; Sessa, Ben, et al (2010). 'The administration of psilocybin to healthy, hallucinogen-experienced volunteers

in a mock-functional magnetic resonance imaging environment: a preliminary investigation of tolerability'. *Journal of Psychopharmacology.*

11. Freud, Sigmund (1940) 'An excerpt from *An Outline of Psychoanalysis*, of which three quarters was written in 1938 but never completed. It was published in 1940, a year after his death. London, Hogarth Press.

12. To end this section on my personal journey, I would like to leave you with a symbolically striking image from the UK's first international conference dedicated entirely to psychedelic research since the early 1960s, Breaking Convention, which I co-chaired with David Luke of Greenwich University and Cameron Adams, Anna Waldstein and David King of Kent University. It was the most wonderful event with 600 delegates from 29 countries and all the glitterati of the international research field gathered together for three days at the University of Kent in Canterbury. There were many memorable moments from that weekend, but for me the pinnacle has to be taking my seat in the opening session looking out over a sea of flowers (we gave everyone a flower as they entered the main hall) and welcoming a new wave of international interest into this fascinating and colourful subject of study. I know of no other topic that can so seamlessly incorporate such disparate disciplines as chemistry, botany, sociology, anthropology, psychology, law, politics, art, design and medicine all under one roof as that of the study of the psychedelic drugs, and I am deeply proud to be part of such a vibrant and progressive community.

Chapter 2: The Experience and the Drugs

1. Adams, Douglas (1979) *The Hitchhikers Guide to the Galaxy.* London: Pan Books.
2. Leary, Timothy (1968) *High Priest.* New York: The New American Library Inc.
3. Lesh, Phil (2005) *Searching for the Sound: My Life with the Grateful Dead.* New York: Little, Brown and Company.
4. Pahnke, Walter N. (1966) 'Drugs and Mysticism'. *The International Journal of Parapsychology*, vol. VIII (no. 2), Spring 1966; 295–313.
5. Griffiths, Roland R., Richards, W. A., McCann, U., Jesse, R. (2006) 'Psilocybin can occasion mystical-type experiences having substantial and sustained personal meaning and spiritual significance.' *Psychopharmacology* (Berl) 187: 268–283.
6. Leary, Timothy (1968) *High Priest.* New York: The New American Library Inc.
7. McKenna, Terence (1982) *Food of the Gods.* London: Bantam Press.
8. Bill Richards, B. and Pahnke, W (1966) 'Implications of LSD and Experimental Mysticism'. *Journal of Religion and Health*, Vol. 5, 1966, 175–208.
9. The Jimi Hendrix Experience. From the album *Are You Experienced?* London: Track Records. I understand from the book *Becoming Jimi Hendrix: From Southern Crossroads to Psychedelic London, the Untold Story of a Musical*

Genius by Steven Roby and Brad Schreiber (De Capo Press, 2010) that until he made his fist guitar at the age of six (which was clearly a transitional object to bridge the passage from a difficult childhood and allow him to express himself), Jimi had an imaginary friend to whom he spoke to a lot of the time. He called this friend 'Cessa' or 'Sessa'. Weird, I know.

10. Leary, Timothy, Ralph Metzner, and Richard Alpert (1963/1992). *The Psychedelic Experience: A Manual Based on the Tibetan Book of the Dead*. New York: Citadel Press.

11. I feel justified to say this from reading the results of Roland Griffith's 2006 experiment in which subjects, with little or no previous experience of psychedelics, spontaneously reported just such an outcome in the majority of cases.

12. Hofmann, Albert. (1979/2005) *LSD My Problem Child: Reflections on Sacred Drugs, Mysticism, and Science*. Sarasota: MAPS.

13. From the song 'Museum' by Donovan Leitch on his 1967 album *Mellow Yellow*.

14. See www.erowid.org, www.bluelight.org, and www.shroomwithaview.org for examples of such drug forums. Well worth a browse.

15. Shulgin, Alexander and Shulgin, Anne. (1991) *PIHKAL: Phenethylamines I Have Known And Loved – A Chemical Love Story*. Berkley: Transform Press.

16. Shulgin, Alexander. and Shulgin, Anne. (1997) *TIHKAL: Tryptamines I Have Known And Loved – A Chemical Love Story*. Berkley: Transform Press.

17. Strassman, Rick. (1995) *DMT: The Spirit Molecule*.

18. Passie, Torsten, Halpern John H, Stichtenoth DO, Emrich HM, Hintzen A (2008). 'The Pharmacology of Lysergic Acid Diethylamide: a Review'. *CNS Neuroscience and Therapeutics* 14 (4): 295–314.

19. Huxley, Aldous. (1954) *The Doors of Perception*. London: Chatto and Windus.

20. Carhart-Harris, Robin et al (2012) 'Psilocybin augments subjective and neural responses to autobiographical memory cues: An fMRI study with implications for psychedelic-assisted psychotherapy'. *British Journal of Psychiatry*. IN PRINT for 2012.

21. Tendler, S. and May, D (1984) *Brotherhood of Eternal Love*. London: Harper Collins.

22. Fielding, Leaf. (2011) *To Live Outside the Law: Caught by Operation Julie, Britain's Biggest Drugs Bust*. London: Serpents Tail.

23. Personally, I find the majority of the designs in this genre of Blotter Art to be hideously cheesy New Age rubbish, but I say this just to playfully annoy my friend Monkey, who holds perhaps the world's largest collection of Blotter Art and whose website is well worth a look. Last year when we held the UK's first psychedelic conference since the 1960s Monkey helped us out by providing the (un-dipped) blotter paper, which we used to make the name tags for the conference delegates. He also auctioned off some rare blotter sheets signed by Tim Leary and gave the proceeds to the conference. Monkey's website can be found at www.blotterart.co.uk

24. Fantegrossi W. E., Woods, J.H. , and Winmge, G. (2004) 'Transient reinforcing effects of phenylisopropylamine and indoealkylamine hallucinogens in rhesus monkeys'. *Behavioural Pharmacology* 15:149–157.

25. Dishotsky, N. I., et al (1971). 'LSD and genetic damage'. *Science* 172 (3982): 431–40.

26. Grof, Stan and Grof, Christina (eds.) (1989). *Spiritual Emergency: When Personal Transformation Becomes a Crisis.* Los Angeles: Tarcher.

27. Stamets, Paul (1996) *Psilocybin Mushrooms of the World: An Identification Guide.* New York: Ten Speed Press.

28. Strassman, Rick (2001) *DMT: The Spirit Molecule.* New York: Park Street Press.

29. Shulgin, Alexander and Shulgin, Anne. (1991) *PIHKAL: Phenethylamines I Have Known And Loved – A Chemical Love Story.* Berkley: Transform Press.

30. Huxley, Aldous (1954) *The Doors of Perception.* London: Chatto and Windus.

31. Peyote buttons have a notoriously terribly bitter taste, described to me by my colleague Dr. David King as 'simply the worst taste ever'.

32. Halpern, John H., Sherwood AR, Hudson, J. I., Yurgelun-Todd, D., Pope H. G. Jr. (2005) 'Psychological and cognitive effects of long-term peyote use among Native Americans'. *Biol Psychi.* 58(8):624-631.

33. Sessa, Ben (2011) 'Can MDMA enhance Trauma-focused psychotherapy?' *Progress in Neurology and Psychiatry.* Volume 15, Issue 6, 4–7.

34. Cole, Jon et al (2002) 'The content of ecstasy tablets: implications for the study of their long-term effects.' *Addiction.* Volume 97, Issue 12, pages 1531–1536

35. Sessa, Ben (2007) Is there a role for MDMA Psychotherapy in the UK?' *Journal of Psychopharmacology.* Vol 21; 220-221

36. Schifano Francisco, Corkery J., Deluca P., Oyefeso A., Ghodse A. H. (2006) 'Ecstasy (MDMA, MDA, MDEA, MBDB) consumption, seizures, related offences, prices, dosage levels and deaths in the UK (1994–2003).' *Journal of Psychopharmacology* 20(3): 456–463

37. Nimmo S. M., Kennedy B. W., Tullett W. M., Blyth A. S., Dougall J. R. (1993) 'Drug-induced hyperthermia'. *Anaesthesia* 48: 892–895

38. Malberg J. E., Seiden L. S. (1998) 'Small changes in ambient temperature causes large changes in 3,4-methylenedioxymethamphetamine (MDMA)-induced serotonin neurotoxicity and core body temperature in the rat.' *J. Neuroscience* 18: 5086–5094

39. Wolff K., Tsapakis E. M., Winstock A. R., Hartley D., Holt D., Forsling M. L., Aitchison K. J. (2006) 'Vasopressin and oxytocin secretion in response to the consumption of ecstasy in a clubbing population'. *Journal of Psychopharmacology* 20(3): 400–410

40. Sessa, Ben, Nutt, David (2007) 'MDMA, politics and medical research: Have we thrown the baby out with the bathwater?' *J Psychopharmacol* 21: 787-791.

41. Sessa, Ben and Nutt, David (2008) 'Reply to letter by Green, Marsden and Fone (2007) about Sessa and Nutt's editorial (MDMA: baby with the bath water) in the November 2007 Journal.' *Journal of Psychopharmacology,* Vol. 22, No. 4, 457-458

42. Schifano Francisco, Oyefeso A., Webb L., Pollard M., Corkery J., Ghodse A. H. (2003) 'Review of deaths related to taking ecstasy, England and Wales, 1997- 2000.' *BMJ* 326: 80-81

43. Ricaurte, George et al (1985) 'Hallucinogenic amphetamine selectively destroys brain serotonin nerve terminals.' *Science,* 229, 986-988.

44. O'Shea, E., Orio, L., Escobedo, I., Sanchez, V., Camarero, J., Green, A. R., et al. (2006) 'MDMA-induced neurotoxicity: long-term effects on 5- HT biosynthesis and the influence of ambient temperature.' *Br J Pharmacol* 148: 778–785.

45. Hatzidimitriou, G., McCann, U. D. , Ricaurte, George (1999) 'Altered Serotonin Innervation Patterns in the Forebrain of Monkeys Treated with (6)3,4-Methylenedioxymethamphetamine 7 Years Previously: Factors Influencing Abnormal Recovery.' *J Neurosci* 19: 5096– 5107.

46. Sabol, K. E., Lew, R., Richards, J. B., Vosmer, G. L., Seiden, L. S. (1996) 'Methylenedioxymethamphetamine-Induced Serotonin Deficits Are Followed by Partial Recovery Over a 52 Week Period. Part I: Synaptosomal Uptake and Tissue Concentrations.' *J Pharmacol Exp Ther* 276: 846–854.

47. Selvaraj, S. et al (2009) 'Brain Serotonin transporter binding in former users of MDMA ('ecstasy').' *British Journal of Psychiatry.* 194: 355-359

48. Stolaroff, Myron (2004) *The Secret Chief Revealed.* Sarasota: MAPS.

49. Greer, George R., Tolbert, R. (1986) 'Subjective reports of the effects of MDMA in a clinical setting.' *Journal of Psychoactive Drugs* 18(4): 319–327

50. Greer, George., Tolbert, R. (1990) 'The therapeutic use of MDMA.' In Peroutka, S. J. (ed.), *Ecstasy: the Clinical, Pharmacological and Neurotoxicological Effects of the Drug MDMA.* Kluwer: Holland

51. Mithoefer, Michael. et al (2010) 'The safety and efficacy of 3,4-methylenedioxymethamphetamineassisted psychotherapy in subjects with chronic, treatment-resistant posttraumatic stress disorder: the first randomized controlled pilot study.' *Journal of Psychopharmacology.* 0(0) 1-14

52. Bergman, S. (1999) 'Ketamine: review of its pharmacology and its use in pediatric anesthesia.' *Anesth Prog.* 46(1): 10–20.

53. Indeed, when ketamine is infused intravenously (as happened to me when I took part in a study with ketamine at the Maudsley Hospital in 2011) the experience wore off fairly soon after Dr. James Stone stopped the syringe pump, leaving me gaping in incredulous disbelief at the hospital surroundings for half an hour before stepping out onto the streets of Peckham in London.

54. Lilly John. (1973) *The Center of the Cyclone* (2nd ed.). London: Bantam Books.

55. Jansen, Karl. (2004) *Ketamine: Dreams and Realities.* Sarasota: MAPS.

56. Moore, Marcia. (1978) *Journeys into the Bright World*. Rockport: Para Research Inc

57. A final note about ketamine is that recent developments in the world of research chemicals (RCs) have spawned methoxetamine, a new ketamine derivative heralded as 'bladder friendly ketamine'. Like all RCs, no one knows about the potential toxicology of this drug.

58. Shulgin, Alexander. and Shulgin, Anne. (1991) *'PIHKAL: Phenethylamines I Have Known And Loved – A Chemical Love Story.'* Berkley: Transform Press.

59. Moya, P.R.; Berg, K.A.; Gutiérrez-Hernandez, M.A., Sáez-Briones, P., Reyes-Parada, M., Cassels, B. K., Clarke, W. P. (2007). 'Functional selectivity of hallucinogenic phenethylamine and phenylisopropylamine derivatives at human 5-hydroxytryptamine (5-HT)2A and 5-HT2C receptors'. *The Journal of pharmacology and experimental therapeutics* 321 (3): 1054–61.

60. Ambrose ,J. B., Bennett, H. D., Lee, H. S., Josephson, S. A. (May 2010). 'Cerebral vasculopathy after 4-bromo-2,5-dimethoxyphenethylamine ingestion'. *The Neurologist* 16 (3): 199–202.

61. Stolaroff, Myron (1994) *Thanatos to Eros – Thirty-Five years of psychedelic exploration.* Berlin: VWB

62. Stolaroff, Myron. (2004 / 1997) The Secret Chief Revealed: Conversations with a pioneer of the underground psychedelic therapy movement. Sarasota: MAPS.

63. Sessa, Ben and Meckel Fischer, Friederike. (2011) 'Underground LSD, MDMA and 2-CB-assisted Individual and Group Psychotherapy in Zurich: Outcomes, Implications and Commentary.' *Journal of Psychopharmacology / Journal of Independent Scientific Committee on Drugs.* (Accepted June 2011, UNDER PEER REVIEW.)

64. Fantegrossi, W. E., Harrington A. W, .Eckler, J. R., Arshad, S., Rabin, R.A., Winter, J. C., Coop, A., Rice, K. C., Woods, J. H .(September 2005). 'Hallucinogen-like actions of 2,5-dimethoxy-4-(n)-propylthiophenethylamine (2C-T-7) in mice and rats.' *Psychopharmacology (Berlin)* 181 (3): 496–503.

65. Theobald, D. S., Staack, R., Puetz, M., Mauer, H. H. (September 2005). 'New designer drug 2,5-dimethoxy-4-ethylthio-β-phenethylamine (2C-T-2): studies on its metabolism and toxicological detection in rat urine using gas chromatography/mass spectrometry'. *J Mass Spectrom.* 2008 Mar ;43(3):305-16.

Chapter 3: Early Pioneers

1. Mitchell, S. Weir, (1896) 'The Effects of Anhelonium Lewinii (the Mescal Button)," *Brit. Med. J.* 2:1625-1629.

2. Ellis, Havelock (1897) 'The phenomena of mescal intoxication'. *The Lancet*, Volume 149, Issue 3849, Pages 1540 - 1542

3. Lewin, Louis. (1894) 'Über Anhalonium Lewinii und andere Cacteen' — On Anhalonium lewinii and other cacti.' *Archiv für Experimentelle Pathologie und Pharmakologie.* 24: 401-411

4. Stoll, Werner A. (1947) 'Lysergsäure-diäthyl-amid, ein Phantastikum aus der Mutterkorngruppe.' *Schweiz Arch Neut.* 60: 279.

5. Heffter, Arthur (1898). 'Ueber Pellote - Beiträge zur chemischen und pharmakologischen Kenntniss der Cacteen Zweite Mittheilung'. *Naunyn-Schmiedeberg's Archives of Pharmacology* 40 (5–6): 385–429

6. Roberts, Andy (2008) *Albion Dreaming: A popular history of LSD in Britain.* London: Marshall Cavendish.

7. Hofmann, Albert. (2005) 'LSD: Problem Child and Wonder Drug.' Sarasota: MAPS.

8. Sandison, Ronald. and Sessa, Ben. (2008) 'An Interview with Dr Ronald Sandison – LSD Pioneer in UK Psychiatry.' *Multidisciplinary Association for Psychedelic Studies Bulletin.* (Autumn Volume, 2008).

9. Sandison, Ronald. A., Spencer, A. M., Whitelaw, J. D. (1954) 'The therapeutic value of LSD in mental illness.' *J Ment Sci.* 1954 Apr;100(419):491-507.

10. http://www.youtube.com/watch?v=Hd4rgyZzseY

11. Busch, A. K., Johnson, W. C. (1950) 'L.S.D. 25 as an aid in psychotherapy'. *Dis. Nerv. System.* 1950 August;11:241

12. Osmond, Humphrey. and Smythies, John. (1952) 'Schizophrenia: A new approach.' *The British Journal of Psychiatry.* 98: 309-315

13. Ludwig, A. (1970) 'LSD treatment in alcoholism.' In Gamage, J. R. & Zerkin, E. L. *Hallucinogenic Drug Research.* Beloit, Wisconsin: Stash Press.

14. Krupitsky, Evgeny. M. (1995) 'Ketamine psychedelic therapy (KPT) of alcoholism and neurosis.' In: H. Leuner (Ed.) *Yearbook of the European College for the Study of Consciousness.* Berlin: Verlag Fur Wissenschaft und Bildung.

15. Alcoholics Anonymous (1984), *"Pass it on": the story of Bill Wilson and how the A.A. message reached the world.* New York: Alcoholics Anonymous World Services, Inc.

16. Huxley, Aldous. (1954) *The Doors of Perception.* London: Chatto and Windus.

17. Lee, M. A. and Shalin, B. (1992) *Acid Dreams. The complete social history of LSD: The CIA, the sixties and beyond.* New York: Grove Press.

18. Huxley, Aldous. (1962) *Island.* New York: Harper and Brothers.

19. Huxley, Aldous. edited by Michael Horowitz and Cynthia Palmer (1999) *Moksha: Aldous Huxley's Classic Writings on Psychedelics and the Visionary Experience.* Vermont: Park Street Press.

20. Grof, Stanislav (2001). *LSD Psychotherapy* (3rd ed.). Sarasota: MAPS.

21. Greenfield, Robert. (2006) *Timothy Leary. A Biography.* Boston: Houghton Mifflin Harcourt

22. Leary, Timothy. (1957). *Interpersonal diagnosis of personality.* New York: Ronald Press.

23. Leary, Timothy. & Metzner, Ralph. (1968). 'Use of psychedelic drugs in prisoner rehabilitation.' *British Journal of Social Psychiatry* Vol. 2: 27-51.

24. Doblin, Rick. (1998) 'Dr. Leary's Concord Prison Experiment: a 34-year follow-up study.' *J Psychoactive Drugs.* 1998 Oct-Dec;30(4):419-26.

25. Hollingshead, Michael (1973) *The Man Who Turned On the World*. New York: Abelard-Schuman Publ. (also Blond & Briggs, Ltd.)

26. Leary, Timothy (1968) *High Priest*.(Second Edition, 1995). Berkeley: Ronin Press.

27. Pahnke, Walter N. (1969) 'Psychedelic drugs and mystical experience.' *Int Psychiatry Clin* 5: 149–162.

28. Doblin, Rick. (1991) 'The Good Friday Experiment - A twenty-five year follow-up and methodological critique.' *Journal of Transpersonal Psychology* Vol. 23 (1): 1-28.

29. Zaehner, R.C. (1972) *Drugs, Mysticism and Make Believe*. London: Collins.

30. Meher Baba (1966) *God in a Pill? On L.S.D. and The High Roads*. Walnut Creek: Sufism Reoriented, Inc.

31. Masters, Robert. L. and Houston, Jean. (1966). *The Varieties of Psychedelic Experience*. Vermont: Park Street Press.

32. Downing, Joseph J., and Wygant, William, Jr. (1964) 'Psychedelic experience and religious belief.' In R. Blum and Associates, editors. *Utopiates: The Use and Users of LSD-25*. New York: Atherton. Pp. 187-198.

33. Clark, W. H. (1974) 'Hallucinogen drug controversy'. In: Radouco-Thomas, S., Villeneuve, A., Radouco-Thomas, C. (eds) *Pharmacology, Toxicology, and Abuse of Psychomimetics (Hallucinogens)*. Quebec: Les Presses de l'Universite' Laval: 411-418.

34. Sandison, Ronald. to Sessa, Ben. (2007) Personal communication.

35. Kast, Eric (1967). 'Attenuation of anticipation: a therapeutic use of lysergic acid diethylamide' *Psychiat. Quart.* 41 (4): 646–57.

36. Grinspoon, Lester. and Bakalar, J. (1979) *Psychedelic Drugs Reconsidered*. New York: The Lindesmith Center.

37. Malleson, Nicolas. (1971) 'Acute Adverse Reactions to LSD in clinical and experimental use in the United Kingdom.' *Br J Psychiatry.* 1971 Feb;118(543):229-30.

38. Laing, Adrian (1997) *R.D. Laing: A Biography*. London: Harper Collins.

39. Laing's influence on clinical psychiatry is legendary. In the early 1990s, when I was twenty-one, I came across his seminal work *The Divided Self* (1960) while I was taking a year out from medicine to complete a psychology degree. At the time, I was all fuelled up with anti-psychiatry sentiments, and I read the book with a mixture of admiration and envy, knowing he wrote it when he was a junior doctor himself, aged just 23. His precise dissecting of the rot and junk that littered psychiatry at the time blew me and my anti-authority student colleagues away.

40. Leary, Timothy. (1980) *The Politics of Ecstasy.* Berkley: Ronin Publishing.

41. Zeal, Paul. (2010) Personal communication.

42. Kyaga, S. et al (2011) 'Creativity and mental disorder: family study of 300 000 people with severe mental disorder.' *British Journal of Psychiatry* November 2011 199:373-379

Chapter 4: The Prehistory and Ancient History of Hallucinogens

1. McKenna, Terence (1982) *Food of the Gods.* London: Bantam Press.
2. For anyone interested in continuing this line of thought I recommend you need look no further than the wonderful 'Lucifer', who travels around in a levitating tepee hosting lectures and presentations from entheogenic speaker-listeners as part of the Portal For The Immortal collective; a group of UK-psychonauts who describe themselves as "an avatar network of higher dimensional beings producing & creating the most profound visions of the higher dimensional realms", which is certainly how it seemed to me when I spoke for them at Sunrise Festival last year and this year.
   Lucifer can be found at http://www.facebook.com/groups/immortalists/
3. Carhart-Harris, Robin. (2012) Personal communication.
4. Gould, Steven Jay (1997) *Evolution: The Pleasures of Pluralism.* The New York Review of Books, June 26, 1997, pp. 47-52.
5. Ramachandran, V.S. (2011) *The Tell-Tale Brain.* William Heinemann, London.
6. Sessa, Ben. (2012) '*The Tell-Tale Brain* by V.S. Ramachandran. Book review.' For the Journal of Neuropsychoanalysis. IN PRINT.
7. There are several important papers of the 1960s that explore the role for psychedelic drugs in understanding and treating autism. These include:
   a. Freedman, A.M. et al (1962) 'Autistic Schizophrenic Children. An Experiment in the Use of D-lysergic acid diethylamide (LSD-25).' *Archives of General Psychiatry,* 1962; 6 (203-213)
   b. Simmons, J. et al (1966) 'Modification of Autistic Behavior with LSD-25.' *American Journal of Psychiatry*, May 1966, pp. 1201-1211
   c. Mogar, R. E., Aldrich, R. W. (1969) 'The use of psychedelic agents with autistic schizophrenic children.' *Behav Neuropsychiatry* 1: 44–50.
8. Griffiths, Roland. (2011) Personal Communication.
9. Another interesting psychedelic fact about elephants: In 1962 a shady US government official working with the CIA, Dr. Louis Jolyon 'Jolly' West injected the pride of Oklahoma Zoo's elephant, Tusko, with a wildly poorly judged dose of LSD using a dart rifle. The beast went into an unremitting epileptic seizure and died an hour and a half later, but not before Dr. West had also pumped formidable quantities of phenobarbitone and chlorpromazine into it. So it is not clear whether Tusko died from the dose of LSD or the heavy sedatives, but West certainly misjudged the dose of the psychedelic, giving Tusko 300mg of LSD. A more accurate dose, given interspecies scaling and the size of an elephant's brain would have been more like one milligram. Rumour has it that Jolly West, who was part of the CIA's MK-ULTRA programme operating in the 1950s to develop LSD as a truth serum for the military, was high on his own supply at the time). This and other fascinating stories of psychedelic history can be found in: Lee, M. A., and Shalin, B. (1992) *Acid Dreams.*

The Complete Social History of LSD: The CIA, the Sixties and Beyond. New York: Grove Press.

10. Eliade, Mercia (1951) *Le Chamanisme et les techniques archaïques de l'extase*, 1951 - *Shamanism: Archaic Techniques of Ecstasy.* Princeton: Princeton University Press.

11. Kehoe, Alice (2000) *Shamans and Religion: An Anthropological Exploration in Critical Thinking. Long* Grove: Waveland Press.

12. Harner, Michael, (1980) *The Way of the Shaman: A Guide to Power and Healing.* New York: Harper & Row.

13. Unfortunately modern Western society does not always recognise the role of shamanic approaches to spirituality. In the UK BBC Radio 4, which likes to represent as wide a range of religions as possible on their morning 'Thought for the Day' slot, has so far not accepted my proposition for a brief sermon on the subject of entheogenic spirituality. Perhaps one day this will change.

14. Schultes, Richard Evans; and Albert Hofmann (1980). *The Botany and Chemistry of Hallucinogens* (2nd ed. ed.). Springfield, Ill.: Thomas.

15. Hofmann, Albert., Wasson, G.R., Ruck, C. and Staples, B. (1998) *The Road to Eleusis: Unveiling the Secret of the Mysteries.* New Castle, PA: Hermes Press.

16. Ruck, Carl. P. and Webster, P. (2006) 'Symposium: The Mythology and Chemistry of the Eleusinian Mysteries.' *Proceedings of the 2006 World Psychedelic Forum conference: LSD.* Basel, Switzerland.

17. Forte, Robert (Editor) (1997) *Entheogens and the Future of Religion.* San Francisco: Council on Spiritual Practices.

18. Allegro, J. M., Irvin, J. R., Ruck, Carl P. (1970) *The Sacred Mushroom and The Cross: A study of the nature and origins of Christianity within the fertility cults of the ancient Near East.* London: Hodder & Stoughton Ltd

19. Merkur, Dan. (2000) The mystery of manna: the psychedelic sacrament of the Bible, Vermont: Inner Traditions / Bear and Co.

20. Deep Purple, (1968) 'Mandrake Root.' From the album *Shades of Deep Purple.*

21. Caporael, L. (1976). 'Ergotism: The Satan loosed in Salem?' *Science, 192* (4234), 21-26

22. Three important books exploring mental illness and its systemic role in society, which were highly influential for me during my medical education:
    a. Szasz, Thamas. (1961) T*he Myth of Mental Illness.* New York: Harper and Row.
    b. Foucault, Michel. (1964) *Madness and Civilisation.* New York: Pantheon Books.
    c. Goffman, Irvin. (1961) *Asylums: Essays on the Social Situation of Mental Patients and Other Inmates.* New York: Anchor Books..

23. Henderson, Bobby (2005). "Open Letter To Kansas School Board". Available at: http://www.venganza.org/about/open-letter/

24. Many people believe the Gong Mythology holds just as much claim as a viable explanation of spiritual truth as does Christianity. It goes briefly as follows: Once upon a time there was a planet out there called Planet Gong, from which

come small green men, the Pot Head Pixies, with propellers on their heads. They zoom around in flying teapots by a process known as 'glidding'. On Planet Gong there is an Angel's Egg, which is someway connected to the Octave Doctors (of which there are 32) — who are the guardians of the Egg. The mystery of Planet Gong is revealed to an ordinary hapless human called Zero the Hero, who, after drinking a special tea, falls asleep and is taken to Planet Gong by the passing Captain Capricorn. Zero later realises he is in fact a specially chosen prophet and his assignment is to save planet Earth from the ignorant human race. Unfortunately during a crucial point in his mission he makes the decision to fraternise with celestial groupies at a great cosmic party rather than build a temple, thereby failing to complete his task - in this life, at least. But all is not lost. After he is dead and in his spiritual form, in 2032, he finally manages to unite the hopeless souls of Earth together in order that they can transcend this life and enter a new enlightened form of consciousness, this saving the planet.

The most important thing about this Gong story — which is the brainchild of the wonderfully spiritually psychedelic visionary Daevid Allen - is that there is a good empirical validity for it; a fine number of albums nonetheless from the international psychedelic band Gong, which have been reproduced all over the world and are regularly worshipped by many captive followers who believe there is nothing less magical and unbelievable in this story than what the Christians tell us about Jesus' direct relation to God. Albums by Gong well worth a listen to illustrate the famous Gong Mythology include: Flying Teapot (1973): Radio Gnome Trilogy, Part 1, Angel's Egg (1973) Radio Gnome Trilogy, Part 2 and You (1974): Radio Gnome Trilogy, Part 3

25. James, William. (1902) *The Varieties of Religious Experience.* London: Longmans, Green and Co.

26. Masters, Robert L. and Houston, Jean. (1966). The Varieties of Psychedelic Experience. Vermont: Park Street Press.

Chapter 5: Hippie Heydays and the Birth of Ecstasy

1. *Withnail and I.* (1987) Directed by Bruce Robinson.

2. Morgan, B. (2006) *I Celebrate Myself: The Somewhat Private Life of Allen Ginsberg.* London: Viking / Penguin.

3. Leary, Timothy. (1968) *High Priest.* New York: The New American Library Inc.

4. Three excellent books to learn about the social history of psychedelia, particularly in the USA:

   a. Lee, M. A. and Shalin, B. (1992) *Acid Dreams. The complete social history of LSD: The CIA, the sixties and beyond.* New York: Grove Press.

   b. Stevens, Jay. (1987) *Storming Heaven: LSD and the American Dream.* New York: Grove Press.

   c. Tendler, S. and May, D (1984) *Brotherhood of Eternal Love.* London: Harper Collins.

5. Kesey, Ken. (1962) *One Flew Over The Cuckoo's Nest.* New York: Viking Press.

6. Kerouac, Jack. (1957) *On The Road.* New York: Viking Press.

7. Wolfe, Tom. (1968) *The Electric Kool-Aid Acid Test.* New York: Farrar, Strous and Giroux.

8. Kripal, J. J. and Shuck, G. W. (2005) *On the Edge of the Future: Esalen and the Evolution of American Culture.* Bloomington: Indiana University Press.

9. *Castaneda, Carlos. (1968) The Teachings of Don Juan: A Yaqui Way of Knowledge.* Berkley: University of California Press.

10. Greenfield, Robert. (2006) Timothy Leary. A Biography. Boston: Houghton Mifflin Harcourt

11. I present a monthly radio show (*'Dr Ben's Psychedelic Love-In presents In The Psychiatrist's Flares'*) with my aurally-lysergic colleagues Chris S. and Rupert M. (producer), which is broadcast throughout Somerset on 105.3 FM and available on the internet at: http://10radio.org/index.php?page= psychedelic-love-in

12. Perry, Charles. (2005) The Haight-Ashbury. New York: Wenner Books.

13. http://www.youtube.com/watch?v=aTgrioOyWEo

14. Miles, Barry. (2005) Hippie. London: Cassell Illustrated /Octopus Publishing Ltd.

15. Neville, Richard. (2012) Hippie Hippie Shake. New York: Overlook TP.

16. Fielding, Leaf. (2011) To Live Outside The Law. London: Serpents Tail.

17. Sessa, Ben. (2012) 'Ecstasy aged 23 years old in the UK: Development Implications for Middle Age.' *The European Journal of Psychiatry and Psychology.* IN PRINT.

18. Shulgin, Alexander and Shulgin, Anne. (1991) 'PIHKAL: Phenethylamines I Have Known And Loved – A Chemical Love Story.' Berkley: Transform Press.

19. Eisner, Bruce. (1989) *Ecstasy: The MDMA Story.* Berkley: Ronin Publishing..

20. In 2000 I travelled around India on my own for six months and – completely unaware what sort of place it was – took the obligatory AIDS test and stayed in the Osho 'intimacy' ashram in Pune for a month. It was beautiful. At that point in my journey, as well as studying meditation, I also learned the double educational message of devotion to, and the importance of questioning, one's guru. Developing my own form of meditation, I spent most of my time lying at the bottom of the swimming pool holding my breath and counting in Hindi; it was too hot to be anywhere else.

21. Colin, M. (1997) *Altered State: The Story of Ecstasy Culture and Acid House.* London: Serpents Tail.

22. I didn't make it out of London for the Castlemorton event, although, as students, we heard about it and wished we were there. But we did make it to the Criminal Justice Bill march and the Reclaim The Streets parties of the mid nineties, which saw ravers dancing up to lines of policemen in scenes reminiscent of the sixties anti-Vietnam marches — or at least that's what we liked to think. At the time, London was awash with warehouse and squat parties — impromptu raves

springing up in the suburbs with the party address not revealed until the last minute over one of the many pirate radio stations. At the peak of it, my flatmate and I serendipitously discovered one such station spinning their vinyl and transmitting in FM from the roof of the block where we lived in Archway. I gather now they all broadcast MP3s from their laptops over the internet, sigh.

23. Top of The Pops was a long-running popular weekly music show in the UK. My friends and I were in the BBC studio the night The Shamen played 'Ebenezer Goode'. We were bopping on the gallery to that one.

24. http://www.maps.org/research/mdma/studies/mp1/

25. Doblin, Rick. (2004) 'Exaggerating MDMA's Risks to Justify A Prohibitionist Policy.' Published on MAPS website: http://www.maps.org/mdma/rd011604.html

26. Sessa, Ben (2005) 'Can psychedelics have a role in psychiatry again?' *British Journal of Psychiatry 186*: 457–459

Chapter 6: Psychedelics and Creativity

1. Sessa, Ben. (2008) 'Is it time to revisit the role of psychedelic drugs in enhancing human creativity?' *J Psychopharmacology*; 22; 821

2. Heilman, K. M., Nadeau, S. E., Beversdorf, D. O. (2003) Creative innovation: possible brain mechanisms.' *Neurocase* 9: 369–379.

3. Zinkhan, G. (1993) 'Creativity in Advertising.' *Journal of Advertising* 22, 2: 1-3.

4. Ede Frecska, Vivien Magyar, Csaba E. Moré, and Luis E. Luna (2011) 'Enhancement of Creative Expression and Entoptic Phenomena as After-Effects of Repeated Ayahuasca Administration.' Submitted to *Journal of Psychopharmacology.* May 2011. Under peer review.

5. Luke, David (2010) Rock art or Rorsarch: Is there more to entopics than meets the eye? Time and Mind: *The Journal of Archaeology, Consciousness and Culture.* Volume 3—Issue 1, pp. 9–28

6. Literary examples of altered states influencing creative writing include:
   a. Coleridge, ST (1816) *Kubla Khan.* New Ed edition (2004) Reading, UK: Two Rivers Press.
   b. Dumas, A (1844) *The Count of Monte Cristo.* Penguin Classics (2003). London: Penguin.
   c. Tennyson, AL (1832) *The Lotus Eaters.* New Ed edition (2000) Oxford, UK: Oxford University Press.

7. Artaud, A (1937) *The Peyote Dance.* (1976) New York: Farrar, Straus and Giroux.

8. Michaux, H (1956) Miserable Miracle. San Francisco: City Lights Books (1963).

9. Chamberline, Dean, and Sessa, Ben and (2007) 'Pictures in psychiatry: Albert Hofmann.' *British J Psychiatry* 190: 1-a2-1.

10. Dobkin de Rios, M, Janiger, Oscar (2003) LSD, *Spirituality and the Creative Process.* Vermont: Park Street Press.

11. Krippner, Stanley (1972) 'Mescaline psilocybin and creative artists.' In: Tart, Charles T., (ed), *Altered States of Consciousness.* New Jersey, USA: John Wiley and Sons.

12. Barron, Frank (1965) 'The Creative Process and the Psychedelic Experience.' *Explorations Magazine.* Berkley, California, June–July.

13. McGlothlin, WH, Cohen, S, McGlothlin, MS (1967) 'Long lasting effects of LSD on normals.' *Arch Gen Psychiatry* 17: 521–532.

14. Harman, W. W., McKim, R. H., Mogar, R. E., Fadiman, James, Stolaroff, Myron J. (1966) 'Psychedelic agents in creative problem solving: a pilot study.' *Psychol Rep* 19: 211–227.

15. Stafford, P.G., Golightly, B.H. (1967) *LSD – the problem-solving psychedelic,* chapter VII. London: Tandom Books, pp. 207–209.

16. Markoff, J. (2006) *What the Dormouse Said: How the Sixties Counter- culture Shaped the Personal Computer Industry.* New York, USA: Penguin Group.

17. Kleps, Art (1967) 'Creative Problem Solving' in *LSD: The problem-solving psychedelic,* chapter III. by Stafford, PG, Golightly, BH (eds),. Award Books: New York p. 46.

Chapter 7: Modern Non-Western Uses of Natural Plant and Fungi Psychedelics

1. Gilk, Paul (2009). *"Green Politics is Eutopian".* Cambridge, UK: The Lutterworth Press.

2. Evans Schultes, Hofmann, Albert and Ratsch, Christian (1998) *Plants of the Gods.* New York: Healing Arts Press.

3. Wasson, R. Gordon (1957) 'Seeking the Magic Mushroom.' *Life magazine,* May 13, 1957

4. Maria Sabina quoted (in translation) in Halifax, J. (1979) Shamanic Voices: A Survey of Visionary Narratives, New York: E.P. Dutton. Pp 203-205. Taken from the tremendous book edited by my friend Robert Forte, *Entheogens and the Future of Religion.* San Francisco: Council on Spiritual Practices.

5. Arthur, James (2003) *Mushrooms and Mankind: The Impact of Mushrooms on Human Consciousness and Religion.* San Diego, CA: The Book Tree.

6. Samorini, G. (2000) *Animals and Psychedelics.* Park Street Press, Rochester, Vermont.

7. Letcher, Andy. (2007) *Shroom: A Cultural History of the Magic Mushroom.* London: Ecco.

8. Letcher, Andy. (2011) Personal communication.

9. Gottlieb, Adam. (1977) *Peyote and other psychoactive cacti.* Berkley: Ronin Publishing.

10. Halpern John H., Sherwood AR, Hudson JI, Yurgelun-Todd D, Pope HG Jr. (2005) 'Psychological and cognitive effects of long-term peyote use among Native Americans.' *Biol Psychi.* 58(8):624-631.

11. Alper, K. and Cordell, G. (2001) *Ibogaine, Volume 56: Proceedings from the First International Conference (The Alkaloids).* Waltham, MA: Academic Press.

12. Ball, M. (2007) Sage Spirit: Salvia Divinorum and the Entheogenic Experience. Oregon: Kyandara Publishing

13. Metzner, Ralph. (2005) *Sacred Vine of Spirits: Ayahuasca.* Vermont: Park Street Press.

14. Burroughs, William S. (1963) *The Yage Letters.* San Francisco: City Lights,.

15. McKenna, T. (1993) *True Hallucinations.* San Francisco: Harper.

16. http://www.guardian.co.uk/politics/2011/sep/05/psychedelic-therapy-war-on-drugs

17. Holland, Julie (Editor) (2010) The Pot Book: A Complete Guide to Cannabis: Its Role in Medicine, Politics, Science, and Culture. Sarasota: MAPS.

18. Holland, J. (Editor) (2001) *Ecstasy: The Complete Guide : A Comprehensive Look at the Risks and Benefits of MDMA.* Park Street Press. New York.

19. Mechoulam, R.; M. Peters, Murillo-Rodriguez (21 Aug 2007). 'Cannabidiol - recent advances'. *Chemistry & Biodiversity* 4 (8): 1678–1692.

20. White, Timothy (2006) *Catch A Fire: The life of Bob Marley.* London: Omnibus Press.

21. Stafford, Peter. (1993) *Psychedelics Encyclopedia.* New York: Ronin Publishing.

22. Evans Schultes, Hofmann and Ratsch (1998) *Plants of the Gods.* New York: Healing Arts Press.

Chapter 8: The Psychedelic Renaissance Part One: Movers and Shakers

1. www.maps.org/psychedelicreview/

2. www.maps.org

3. www.heffter.org

4. www.beckleyfoundation.org

5. www.csp.org

6. www.gaiamedia.org

7. www.horizonsnyc.org

8. I have such happy memories of the event, not least because of the manner in which we put it together: twelve months of endless email chains and Skype meetings (I counted over 10,000 messages in all) between Anna, Cam, myself and the Daves, and last minute scrabbling for money to put together the necessary material. It all finalized in hurriedly stuffing 600 conference bags with goodies and making nametags out of (un-dipped) acid blotter paper the evening before the conference in Cameron's house in Canterbury, drinking home brew cider. It was all worth it for a magical weekend coming-together of UK and international psychedelic communities. I knew we had got it right when veteran psychedelic researcher Roland Griffiths came up to me in the bustle of the opening party and said, 'Hey man, this is a great vibe. It reminds me of the Berkley campus in 1965!'

   Check out: www.breakingconvention.org

9. www.stichtingopen.nl

10. www.erowid.org

11. www.bluelight.ru

12. www.shroomwithaview.com

13. www.neurosoup.com

14. Sessa, Ben. (2008) 'Self-medication of LSD and MDMA to treat mental disorders: A case series' in The *Neurosoup Yearly Review 2008*. Neurosoup Trust.

15. www.realitysandwich.com

16. http://www.facebook.com/pages/Regeneration/263070140438485

17. Thanks to Adrian Zieniewicz, director of Psychedelic Spirituality for this brief description of this Facebook Website. Details of how to find them here: http://www.facebook.com/psychedelicspirituality

18. www.ssdp.org

19. Forgive me for omitting anyone from this alphabetically listed section. If you are not on this list, it does not diminish your importance but rather illustrates my ignorance and certainly reflects my greater knowledge of European, especially British, over American professionals.

20. Sessa, Ben and Meckel Fischer, F. (2011) Underground LSD, MDMA and 2-CB-assisted Individual and Group Psychotherapy in Zurich: Outcomes, Implications and Commentary. *Journal of Psychopharmacology / Journal of Independent Scientific Committee on Drugs*. (Accepted June 2011, pending editorial revisions.)

21. Holland, Julie (2010) *Weekends at Belleview*. New York: Random House, Inc,

22. Letcher, Andy. (2007) *Shroom: A Cultural History of the Magic Mushroom*. London: Ecco.

23. Parrott AC, Gibbs A, Scholey AB, King R, Owens K, Swan P, Ogden E, Stough C (2012). 'MDMA and methamphetamine: some paradoxical negative and positive mood changes in an acute dose laboratory study'. *Psychopharmacology (Berl)*. 215(3):527-36.

24. Hintzen, A and Passie, T. (2010) *The Pharmacology of LSD: A critical review*. Oxford University Press, USA and Beckley Foundation, UK. I subsequently wrote a book review of Hintzen and Passie's book, which appeared in the *British Journal of Psychiatry*: Sessa, Ben (2011) 'The Psychopharmacology of LSD by Annalie Hintzen and Torsten Passie. A Book Review' for *The British Journal of Psychiatry*. 199:258-259

25. Ricaurte George A, Yuan J, Hatzidimitriou G, Cord BJ, McCann UD (2002) 'Severe Dopaminergic Neurotoxicity in Primates After a Common Recreational Dose Regimen of MDMA ("Ecstasy").' *Science 297: 2260-3.*

26. Ricaurte George A, Yuan J, Hatzidimitriou G, Cord BJ, McCann UD (2003B) 'Retraction.' *Science 301: 1429.*

27. Roberts, Andy. (2008) *Albion Dreaming: A popular history of LSD in Britain*. London: Marshall Cavendish.

28. Roberts, Thomas B. (2006) *Psychedelic Horizons*. Charlottesville, VA: Imprint Academic.

29. Sewell RA, Halpern JH, Pope HG Jr. (2006) 'Response of cluster headache to psilocybin and LSD.' *Neurology* 27;66: 1920-1922.

30. Strassman, Rick (2001) *DMT: The Spirit Molecule,* New York: Park Street Press.

Chapter 9: The Psychedelic Renaissance Part Two: Contemporary Research

1. Crockford, R.M. (2007) 'LSD in Prague: A Long-Term Follow-Up Study.' *MAPS Bulletin* - volume xvii - number 1 - spring/summer 2007
2. Ng, R. (2008) *Drugs: From Discovery to Approval.* London: Wiley-Blackwell.
3. Michael C. Mithoefer, Mark T. Wagner, Ann T. Mithoefer, Lisa Jerome and Rick Doblin (2010) 'The safety and efficacy of ±3,4-methylenedioxymethamphetamine -assisted psychotherapy in subjects with chronic treatment-resistant posttraumatic stress disorder: the first randomised controlled pilot study.' *Journal of Psychopharmacology*, 19th July 2010
4. www.maps.org/research/mdma
5. Sessa Ben, Nutt David J. (2007) MDMA, politics and medical research: Have we thrown the baby out with the bathwater? *J Psychopharmacol* 21: 787-791
6. Holland, Julie (Editor) (2001) *Ecstasy: The Complete Guide : A Comprehensive Look at the Risks and Benefits of MDMA.* New York: Park Street Press.
7. Agarval, A.K. and Andrade, C (1997) 'Indian Psychiatrists' Attitudes Towards Electroconvulsive Therapy.' *Indian Journal of Psychiatry. 1997, 39 (i) 54-66*
8. http://www.maps.org/media/view/can_ecstasy_help_treat_autism/
9. Alicia Danforth from the Institute of Transpersonal Psychology has produced an interesting study of the history of psychedelic drugs to treat symptoms of autism, which she presented at the MAPS Psychedelic Science conference in San Jose in 2010. Available at: http://www.maps.org/videos/source2/video5.html
10. http://www.maps.org/news-letters/v16n2-html/lsd_swiss.html
11. Kast, Eric (1967). 'Attenuation of anticipation: a therapeutic use of lysergic acid diethylamide.' *Psychiat. Quart.* 41 (4): 646–57.
12. Sewell RA, Halpern JH, Pope HG Jr. (2006) 'Response of cluster headache to psilocybin and LSD.' *Neurology* 27;66: 1920-1922.
13. http://ck-wissen.de/ckwiki/images/1/14/IHS_IHC_2009_BOL_Halpern.pdf
14. Moreno FA, Wiegand CB, Taitano EK, Delgado PL. (2006). 'Safety, tolerability, and efficacy of psilocybin in 9 patients with obsessive-compulsive disorder'. *Journal of Clinical Psychiatry* 67 (11): 1735–40.
15. Grob Charles S., Danforth Alicia L., Chopra GS, Hagerty M, McKay CR, Halberstadt AL, Greer George R. (2011) Pilot study of psilocybin treatment for anxiety in patients with advanced-stage cancer. *Arch Gen Psychiatry.* 2011 Jan;68(1):71-8. Epub 2010 Sep 6.
16. Griffiths, Roland R., Richards, William A., McCann, U, Jesse, Robert (2006) 'Psilocybin can occasion mystical experiences having substantial and sustained personal meaning and spiritual significance.' *Psychopharmacology (Berl)* 187: 268–283.

17. McClean, A., Johnson, W. and Griffiths, Roland. (2011) 'Mystical Experiences Occasioned by the Hallucinogen Psilocybin Lead to Increases in the Personality Domain of Openness.' *J Psychopharmacol* 26 (3)

18. Carhart-Harris Robin L., Erritzoe D, Williams T, Stone JM, Read LJ, Colasanti A, et al. (2012) 'Neural correlates of the psychedelic state as determined by fMRI studies with psilocybin.' *Proc Natl Acad Sci* vol. 109 no. 6 2138-2143

19. Carhart-Harris, Robin. et al (2012) 'Implications for psychedelic-assisted psychotherapy: functional magnetic resonance imaging study with psilocybin.' *BJP* 200:238-244.

20. Strassman RJ, Qualls C, Berg LM. (1996) 'Differential tolerance development to biological and subjective effects of four closely-spaced administrations of N,N-dimethyltryptamine in humans'. *Biological Psychiatry* 39:784-795, 1996

21. Daumann J, Heekeren K, Neukirch A, Thiel CM, Möller-Hartmann W, Gouzoulis-Mayfrank E. (2008) Pharmacological modulation of the neural basis underlying inhibition of return (IOR) in the human 5-HT(2A) agonist and NMDA antagonist model of psychosis. *Psychopharmacology (Berl).* 2008 Nov;200(4):573-83. Epub 2008 Jul 24.

22. Fontanilla et al., (2009) 'The Hallucinogen N,N-Dimethyltryptamine (DMT) Is an Endogenous Sigma-1 Receptor Regulator.' *Science.* 323 (5916): 934-941

23. http://www.ayahuasca.com/science/the-scientific-investigation-of-ayahuasca-a-review-of-past-and-current-research/)

24. Pinto, J.P. (2010) Estudo sobre alterações neurofuncionais após ingestão de ayahuasca. Dissertação de Mestrado em Medicina. Universidade de São Paulo, Ribeirão Preto.

25. Available at: http://www.neip.info/html/objects/_downloadblob.php?cod_blob=1003

26. Dobkin de Rios, M.. and Grob, Charles S. (2005) 'Ayahuasca use in cross-cultural perspective: an introduction.' *Journal of Psychoactive Drugs* 37:119-121.

27. Mabit, J (2007) Ayahuasca in the treatment of addiction. Chapter 6; In *Hallucinogens and Health : New Evidence for Psychedelic Substances as Treatment (Vol 2)* Ed. MJ. Winkelman & TB. Roberts; Westport, Connecticut: Greenwood Publishing Group; pp 87-105.

28. Hancock, Graham (2005). *Supernatural: Meetings with the Ancient Teachers of Mankind*. London: Century.

29. The NHS Information Centre. Statistics on alcohol 2010. http://www.ic.nhs.uk/pubs/alcohol10

30. Miller WR, Wilbourne PL. (2002) 'Mesa Grande: a methodological analysis of clinical trials of treatments for alcohol use disorders'. *Addiction.* Mar;97(3):265-77.

31. Mann K, Lehert K, Morgan M. (2004) 'The efficacy of acamprosate in the maintenance of abstinence in alcohol-dependent individuals: results of a meta-analysis.' *Alcohol Clin Exp Res.* 2004;28:51–63.

32. Srisurapanont et al (2005) 'Naltrexone for the treatment of alcoholism: a meta-analysis of Randomized Controlled Trials'. *Int J. Neuropsychopharmacology;* 2005 Jun;8(2):267-80.

33. Anton, RF (2006) 'Combined pharmacotherapies and behavioral interventions for alcohol dependence.' *JAMA.* 2006 Oct 11;296(14):1727

34. Krupitsky EM, Grinenko AY (1997). 'Ketamine psychedelic therapy (KPT): a review of the results of ten years of research'. *Journal of Psychoactive Drugs* 29 (2): 165–83

35. Krupitsky EM, Burakov AM, Dunaevsky IV, Romanova TN, Slavina TY, Grinenko AY (March 2007). 'Single versus repeated sessions of ketamine-assisted psychotherapy for people with heroin dependence'. *Journal of Psychoactive Drugs* 39 (1): 13–9

36. Jovaisa T, Laurinenas G, Vosylius S, Sipylaite J, Badaras R, Ivaskevicius J (2006). 'Effects of ketamine on precipitated opiate withdrawal'. *Medicina* 42 (8): 625–34.

37. D'Souza, D.C. et al (2012) 'Glycine Transporter Inhibitor Attenuates the Psychotomimetic Effects of Ketamine in Healthy Males: Preliminary Evidence.' *Neuropsychopharmacology* 37, 1036-1046;

38. Correll GE, Futter GE (2006). 'Two case studies of patients with major depressive disorder given low-dose (subanesthetic) ketamine infusions'. *Pain Medicine* 7 (1): 92–5

39. Zarate CA, Singh JB, Carlson PJ, *et al.* (August 2006). 'A randomized trial of an N-methyl-D-aspartate antagonist in treatment-resistant major depression'. *Archives of General Psychiatry* 63 (8): 856–64.

40. Alper, K.R., Beal, D. and Kaplan, C.D., (2001) 'A contemporary history of ibogaine in the United States and Europe. The Alkaloids'. *Chemistry and Biology* 56, 249-281

41. K.R. Alper, H.S. Lotsof, G.M. Frenken , D.J. Luciano , J. Bastiaans (1999). 'Treatment of Acute Opioid Withdrawal with Ibogaine'. *The American Journal on Addictions* 8 (3): 234–42.).

42. http://www.maps.org/research/ibogaine/

43. Mash, D. et al (2000) 'Ibogaine: Complex Pharmacokinetics, Concerns for Safety, and Preliminary Efficacy Measures. Neurobiological Mechanisms of Drugs of Abuse.' *Ann N Y Acad Sci* 2000;914:394-401

44. Sessa, Ben and Meckel Fischer, Friederike (2012)' Underground LSD, MDMA and 2-CB-assisted Individual and Group Psychotherapy in Zurich: Outcomes, Implications and Commentary.' *Journal of Psychopharmacology / Journal of Independent Scientific Committee on Drugs.* (Accepted June 2011, In Press.)

Chapter 10: Psychedelics Caught in the Crossfire of the War on Drugs

1. One such hard-working organisation concerned with fighting against the War on Drugs is the international Students For Sensible Drug Policy. www.ssdp.org

2. www.beckleyfoundation.org

3. EMCDDA (2009) European Monitoring Centre for Drugs and Drug Addiction. Annual report on the state of the drugs problem in Europe, Lisbon.

4. Sessa, Ben (2012) Ecstasy aged 23 years old in the UK: Development Implications for Middle Age. *The European Journal of Psychiatry and Psychology.* IN PRINT.

5. Sessa, Ben and Nutt, David J. (2007) 'MDMA, Politics and Medical Research: Have we thrown the baby out with the bathwater?' *Journal of Psychopharmacology.* Vol. 21: 787-791.

6. Office of National Statistics (2002) – 'Deaths related to drug poisoning in England and Wales 1993–2000 and 1998–2002.' *Health Statistic Quarterly,* Spring 2003 and Spring 2004

7. Halpern, John et al (2004). 'Residual neuropsychological effects of illicit 3,4-methylenedioxymethamphetamine (MDMA) in individuals with minimal exposure to other drugs.' *Drug and Alcohol Dependence* 75 (2004) 135–147

8. Salvaraj, S. et al (2009) 'Brain serotonin transporter binding in former users of MDMA ('ecstasy').' *The British Journal of Psychiatry.* 194: 355-359

9. Huizink, A. et al (2006) 'Symptoms of anxiety and depression in childhood and use of MDMA: prospective, population based study.' *BMJ,* doi: 10.1136/bmj.38743.539398.3A,

10. Nutt, David J. et al (2007) 'The Development of a rational scale to assess the harm of drugs of potential misuse.' *The Lancet* Vol 369:1047-1053

11. http://www.drugscience.org.uk/

12. www.dancesafe.org

13. http://www.maps.org/news-letters/v18n3/v18n3-39to44.pdf

14. Marlatt, G. Alan (2002). *Highlights of Harm Reduction. Harm Reduction: Pragmatic Strategies for Managing High-Risk Behaviors.* London: Guilford Press.

15. Gable, R. S. (2006). 'Acute toxicity of drugs versus regulatory status'. In J. M. Fish (Ed.),*Drugs and Society:* U.S. Public Policy, pp.149-162, Lanham, MD: Rowman & Littlefield Publishers.

16. http://niu.academia.edu/ThomasRoberts/Talks/66495/Looking_Forward_Campus_and_a_Company_powerpoints

17. Roberts, Thomas B. (2006) Psychedelic Horizons. Charlottesville: Imprint Academic.

Bibliography and Further Reading

The books with an asterisk are my particular favourite 'must read' texts for an introduction on the subject of psychedelic drugs.

Arthur, James (2003) *Mushrooms and Mankind: The Impact of Mushrooms on Human Consciousness and Religion*. San Diego: The Book Tree.

Ball, M. (2007) *Sage Spirit: Salvia Divinorum and the Entheogenic Experience*. Oregon: Kyandara Publishing

Burroughs, William. (1963) *The Yage Letters*. San Francisco: City Lights.

Castaneda, Carlos (1968) *The Teachings of Don Juan: A Yaqui Way of Knowledge*. Berkeley: University of California Press.

Dobkin de Rios, and M, Janiger, (2003) *LSD, Spirituality and the Creative Process*. Rochester, Vermont: Park Street Press.

Eliade, Mircea (1951) *Shamanism: Archaic Techniques of Ecstasy*. Princeton: Princeton University Press.

Evans Schultes, Hofmann, Albert and Ratsch, Christian (1998) *Plants of the Gods*. New York: Healing Arts Press.

Fielding, Leaf. (2011) To Live Outside The Law. London: Serpents Tail.

Foucault, M. (1964) Madness and Civilisation. New York: Pantheon Books.

Goffman, I. (1961) *Asylums: Essays on the Social Situation of Mental Patients and Other Inmates*. New York: Anchor Books.

Gottlieb, Adam. (1977) *Peyote and other psychoactive cacti*. New York: Ronin.

Greenfield, Robert. (2006) *Timothy Leary. A Biography*. Boston: Houghton Mifflin Harcourt

*Grinspoon, Lester. and Bakalar, J. (1979) *Psychedelic Drugs Reconsidered*. New York: The Lindesmith Center.

*Grob, Charles – Editor (2002) *Hallucinogens: A Reader*. New York: Tarcher-Putnam.

*Grof, Stanislav (2001). *LSD Psychotherapy* (3rd ed.). Sarasota: MAPS.

Hancock, Graham (2005). *Supernatural: Meetings with the Ancient Teachers of Mankind*. London: Century.

Harner, Michael, *The Way of the Shaman: A Guide to Power and Healing*, New York: Harper & Row.

*Hofmann, A. (1979 / 2005) *LSD My Problem Child: Reflections on Sacred Drugs, Mysticism, and Science*. Sarasota: MAPS.

Hofmann, A., Wasson, G.R., Ruck, C. and Staples, B. *(1998) The Road to Eleusis: Unveiling the Secret of the Mysteries*. New Castle, PA: Hermes Press.

*Holland, Julie. (Editor) (2001) *Ecstasy: The Complete Guide : A Comprehensive Look at the Risks and Benefits of MDMA.* New York: Park Street Press.

Holland, Julie. (Editor) (2010) *The Pot Book: A Complete Guide to Cannabis: Its Role in Medicine, Politics, Science, and Culture.* Sarasota: MAPS.

Hollingshead, Michael (1973) *The Man Who Turned On the World.* New York: Abelard-Schuman.

*Huxley, Aldous. (1954) *The Doors of Perception.* London: Chatto and Windus.

*Huxley, Aldous. (1962) *Island.* New York: Harper and Brothers.

*Huxley, Aldous (Edited by Michael Horowitz and Cynthia Palmer) (1999) *Moksha: Aldous Huxley's Classic Writings on Psychedelics and the Visionary Experience.* New York: Park Street Press.

James, William. (1902) *The Varieties of Religious Experience.* Harlow, UK: Longmans, Green and Co.

Jansen, Karl. (2004) *Ketamine: Dreams and Realities.* Sarasota: MAPS.

Kehoe, Alice (2000) *Shamans and Religion: An Anthropological Exploration in Critical Thinking.* Long Grove: Waveland Press.

Kerouac, Jack. (1957) *On The Road.* New York: Viking Press.

Kesey, Ken. (1962) *One Flew Over The Cuckoo's Nest.* New York: Viking Press.

Laing, Adrian (1997) *R.D. Laing: A Biography.* London: Harper Collins.

Laing, RD (1963) *The Divided Self.* London: Penguin.

Leary, Timothy. (1968) *High Priest.* The New American Library Inc. New York.

*Leary, Timothy; Ralph Metzner, and Richard Alpert (1963/1992). *The Psychedelic Experience: A Manual Based on the Tibetan Book of the Dead* (paperback ed.). New York: Citadel Press.

*Lee, MA and Shalin, B (1992) *Acid Dreams. The complete social history of LSD: The CIA, the sixties and beyond.* New York: Grove Press.

Lesh, Phil. (2005) *Searching for the Sound: My Life with the Grateful Dead.* New York: Little, Brown and Company.

*Letcher, Andy. (2007) *Shroom: A Cultural History of the Magic Mushroom.* London: Ecco.

Lilly John. (1972) *The Center of the Cyclone.* London: Bantam Books.

*Masters, R.L. and Houston, J. (1966). *The Varieties of Psychedelic Experience.* Rochester, Vermont: Park Street Press.

McKenna, Terence. (1993) *True Hallucinations.* San Francisco: Harper

*McKenna, Terence. (1982) *Food of the Gods.* London, Bantam Press.

Merkur, D. (2000) *The mystery of manna: the psychedelic sacrament of the Bible.* New York: Inner Traditions / Bear and Co.

Metzner, Ralph. (2005) *Sacred Vine of Spirits: Ayahuasca.* New York: Park Street Press.

Miles, Barry. (2005) *Hippie.* London: Cassell Illustrated /Octopus Publishing Ltd.

Moore, M. (1978) *Journeys into the Bright World.* Rockport: Para Research Inc

Morgan, Bill. (2006) *I Celebrate Myself: The Somewhat Private Life of Allen Ginsberg.* London: Viking / Penguin.

Neville, R. (2012) Hippie Hippie Shake. New York: Overlook TP.

Perry, Charles. (2005) The Haight-Ashbury. New York: Wenner Books.

*Roberts, Andy (2008) *Albion Dreaming: A popular history of LSD in Britain.* London: Marshall Cavendish.

*Roberts, Thomas B. (2006) *Psychedelic Horizons.* Charlottesville: Imprint Academic.

Samorini, G. (2000) *Animals and Psychedelics.* Rochester, Vermont: Park Street Press.

Schultes, Richard Evans; and Albert Hofmann (1980). *The Botany and Chemistry of Hallucinogens* (2nd ed. ed.). Springfield, Ill.: Thomas.

*Shulgin, Alexander and Shulgin, Anne. (1991) *PIHKAL: Phenethylamines I Have Known And Loved – A Chemical Love Story.* Berkley: Transform Press.

*Shulgin, Alexander and Shulgin, Anne. (1997) *TIHKAL: Tryptamines I Have Known And Loved – A Chemical Love Story.* Berkley: Transform Press.

Stafford, Peter. (1993) *Psychedelics Encyclopedia.* New York: Ronin Publishing.

*Stevens, Jay. (1987) *Storming Heaven: LSD and the American Dream.* New York: Grove Press.

Stolaroff, Myron. (1994) *Thanatos to Eros – Thirty-Five years of psychedelic exploration.* Berlin: VWB.

*Stolaroff, Myron. (2004 / 1997) *The Secret Chief Revealed: Conversations with a pioneer of the underground psychedelic therapy movement.* Sarasota: MAPS.

*Strassman, Rick (2001) *DMT: The Spirit Molecule.* New York: Park Street Press.

Szasz, Thomas. (1961) *The Myth of Mental Illness.* New York: Harper and Row.

Tendler, S. and May, D (1984) *Brotherhood of Eternal Love.* London: Harper Collins.

White, Timothy. (2006) *Catch a Fire: The Life of Bob Marley.* London: Omnibus Press.

Wolfe, Thomas. (1968) *The Electric Kool-Aid Acid Test.* New York: Farrar, Strous and Giroux.

Zaehner, R.C. (1972) *Drugs, Mysticism and Make Believe.* London: Collins.

Index